IF YOU KNEW SUZY

Pushing Past the Boundaries of *Never*

JANE FISCHER
WITH CAROL ANN ROSS

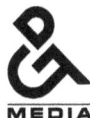

&
MEDIA

MEDIA

Published 2024 by Gildan Media LLC
aka G&D Media
www.GandDmedia.com

Front cover design by David Rheinhardt of Pyrographx

Interior design by Meghan Day Healey of Story Horse, LLC

Library of Congress Cataloging-in-Publication Data is available upon request

ISBN: 978-1-7225-0710-7

10 9 8 7 6 5 4 3 2 1

*To my darling daughter Suzy,
who every day teaches me and everyone she meets
the meaning of endurance, the value of selflessness,
the power of kindness, and the essence of love.*

CONTENTS

Contents

FOREWORD

Jane Fischer's lifelong dream has been to share Suzy's story with the world in order to speak to other parents and families raising children with significant, complex disabilities. Jane's dedication and conviction express the essence of Suzy's strength to overcome her challenges and setbacks.

Suzy and Jane share a trust, a reliance, and a union that eludes words. Suzy's survival and triumphs are a direct outgrowth of Jane's quiet yet powerful insistence on sustaining and enhancing Suzy's life. These two are unafraid to dream, and when it comes to Suzy, no one dreams more intently than Jane.

Where does Jane's energy come from? She would credit Suzy; Suzy would credit Jane. Therein lies the story, one based on the purity of unconditional love and unrelenting hopefulness. Jane pushes on, never becoming a victim, never complaining, never accepting *never*. Suzy mirrors her mom, her greatest teacher. Jane's heart remains huge. Her head remains focused.

Al, Suzy's dad, has been an unceasing workaholic. A different man may have easily caved under the tension and pressure of Suzy's life, under his often necessary position of remaining on the second shelf as Jane tended to Suzy. But this father, husband, and grandpa stayed on course, sometimes questioning, sometimes perhaps wishing he could be the only one in the room with Jane, but always remaining anchored and steadfast on the Fischer turf.

Suzy's two siblings, Beth and Ben, evoke similar admiration. Among Suzy's earliest teachers, champions, and cheerleaders, they are now adults with children of their own, whom they teach to love and understand Aunt Suzy. Although Jane and Al made every attempt to balance the scales, the trajectory of Beth's and Ben's lives was impacted by sharing family life with a sister facing a disability, who has brought them great pleasure, great triumphs, extra responsibility, many defining moments, and difficult burdens. Both Beth and Ben are among Suzy's true heroes. They both chose partners who would also unconditionally accept and love Suzy.

Dear reader, I hope you will feel inspired by Suzy's triumphs and realize the strength each one of us has within.

• • •

Sharon Toriello, MA, LPC was a teacher, a director of guidance, the NJ Principal of the Year in 2004, and Director of Special Education in Livingston, NJ.

PROLOGUE

Suzy's life has been a series of "nevers."

She was born with a quarter of her cerebellar vermis and a malformed brain stem, so the neurologists said she would never learn the simplest tasks. They predicted she would never walk or talk. She would never have a job, never live alone, never have relationships. My husband and I both carried a gene, which we were unaware of, that caused our baby girl to be born with the very rare Joubert syndrome, which prevents the brain from developing normally.

Every specialist we visited had the same advice for us: Suzy was doomed by their prognostications. But I was not, nor would I let this beautiful baby succumb to any doomsday theories. So I began my quest to ensure that my daughter would have every chance at the best life that I could provide. This is the story of her journey, the trials and tribulations, the successes, and the failures. This is a story of the power of perseverance, unwavering support, and most of all love.

The medical community has spoken of rewriting textbooks to accommodate the miraculous achievements Suzy accomplished. She confounded worldwide experts. But she was acutely aware that she would never be able to hold an infant in her arms, and with her natural abundance of nurturing and love, this has left a great hole in her heart.

One day, when we were looking at photos of my niece's baby, I looked up at Suzy, who had a wistful gaze, and said, "You know what, Suze? I have an idea. How would you like it if we wrote a book about your life? We could describe your birth and all the infant stimulation you endured. We can go through your achievements and schooling, the prizes you won, your health challenges, your loving family, and of course our very special relationship. This book will be your baby to cherish forever."

Suzy looked over at me, astonished at my suggestion. She lowered her eyes, and I could feel the processing inside her mind that was always hard for her. In a very quiet voice, she raised her gaze, put her arms around my neck, and replied. "Mommy, that seems like a great idea." She turned and went looking for her companion, yelling, "Jola! My mother is going to write a book about me. Can you believe it! It's going to be like my own baby!"

I peeked around my office door and watched Suzy and Jola exuberantly singing and prancing. My beautiful forty-eight-year-old daughter, who had survived many years more than she was supposed to, who had defied medical journals, had brought so much love to so many: I couldn't think of anyone I knew personally who deserved a testament more than she did. I had opened the door to a fantastic adventure.

Suzy has always understood the world around her in an uncanny way. With her compromised neurological functions, she is unable to understand many abstract concepts, but she can always recognize what people are doing in their lives. With her uncluttered brain and the purity of her spirit, she is the perfect example of what humanity should be. When she stands beside you, you feel her kindness and authentic compassion billow through your body. When she says something tender and warm in her warbling speech, you are enveloped by emotions that make you want to hug her to you and tell her how much you love her. When she looks at you with her sideways gaze, you see in her eyes the absence of emotional contamination that exists in most of us. This is the Suzy effect, and she has it on everyone she meets.

It is so easy to love her, and everyone does. With all the pain and grief she has suffered, she has never lost her optimism or her gentleness. Her mischievousness is still alive, looking for opportunities to make friends and strangers laugh and smile. Suzy is a happy woman who wants to share this happiness and her story with all of humankind.

1

YOU AND ME AGAINST THE WORLD

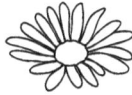

Al and I met in our graduating class at Adelphi University in Garden City, New York.

On our first date, Al, beautifully dressed and sporting a pair of leather driving gloves, picked me up in his sparkling green Corvette. This suave, good-looking man placed me in the front seat of his car and told me my job was to change the radio station. As I moved the knob from a station playing "Sunshine of Your Love" to another playing "California Dreaming," I looked over at him in awe.

Al was attentive and caring, and would surprise me in my dorm room with delicious meals when I couldn't eat the college food. He sent me love notes filled with quotes from the most romantic poems. Although my family was highly educated and sophisticated, his worldliness intrigued me, and I clung to every word of his many tales. He was magnetic, and I was starstruck. Al knew the way to impress me and my brothers. He charmed my parents with his gentlemanly poise when he asked for permission to marry me.

When the time came for him to propose, I was more than ready to say yes. He asked me to help him put tobacco in his pipe. When I told him I couldn't push the leaves into the bulb because there was an object in the way, he laughed and told me I should fish it out. There sat the prettiest diamond I had ever seen. As my eyes glistened with the reflection of the stone, he asked me to spend the rest of my life with him. I wore it proudly. I was the envy of every girl I knew, having snagged a winner.

My mother and father were exemplary parents, who doted on their only daughter and two sons. One might say that their love was unconditional and limitless. One might also say they coddled me, leaving me ill-prepared for adversity. My mother and father always treated me like their baby doll, mother dressing me in crinoline skirts, with my hair parted down the middle in two braids. My father adored his wife and children, giving us a secure and safe existence. Such was my childhood, filled with innocence, happiness, and naivety. I grew up with the expectation that this seamless version of life was the norm.

Al stepped into the shoes of Prince Charming. He was educated, spoke distinctly, looked sporty and fit. Most, of all he loved me and never stopped telling me so. Giddy with excitement, I chose a charmeuse bridal gown, imagining my father by my side. The dress had a waistline so tiny that I must have starved myself to fit into it. I still have it somewhere in a storage closet.

My wedding to Al was a huge, lavish affair. There must have been 250 guests, most of whom I had never seen before. I hardly remember the details, but I do recall my face feeling frozen and fatigued from smiling at all the well-wishers.

I was attractive, slim, meek, and sweet. I took cooking lessons so I could prepare healthy meals for my husband. My mother gave me advice on how to be a doting wife, and my father suggested that I allow Al to manage the finances. If it worked that way for them, I was sure it would work for me too.

We were married on June 28, 1970, when I was twenty-two. Al was in the National Guard at that time and only had a forty-eight-hour pass, so after the wedding, we went to stay at the Plaza Hotel in New York City before he had to go back to serve.

One month later we were hit with terrible news concerning my father. He had just received the test results from his doctor saying that a cancer had metastasized all over his body. In those days, the doctors lacked straightforwardness, and we hopped between hope and honesty. We withheld the harsh truth from my father and probably ourselves, feeding him optimism while my mother fed him healing foods. She believed in the power of unconventional diets.

Watching my father suffer through chemotherapy, with the myriad of relentless side effects, was my first initiation into the future I would have, although I didn't know it then. I did know that my rock, our adored patriarch, was dying too early, and the grief was suffocating. When he passed away nine months later, the void he left was insurmountable. He was only fifty-nine, and his widow, my mother, was fifty-two. The loss was overwhelming to me. I ran to be with my mother at every opportunity, and in retrospect, put her well-being in front of my marriage.

The unexpected swiftness of my own pregnancy added to the complexities of my grief. At only twenty-two years old, with a brand-new job as a teacher, I longed for my father to witness the joys of grandparenthood. My father had been a solid man, who taught kindness and decency. He would proclaim that his children were his greatest investment. When he left us, he left behind unrealized dividends. He existed in my memories like a rhythmic refrain.

Amidst my sorrow, I found myself grappling with the upcoming birth of our daughter. Beth was born after a long and difficult labor. She was a beautiful baby, with a full head of hair and pouty lips that looked as if someone had painted pink lipstick around the edges. She was the first grandchild on both sides of the family, so her arrival brought much joy to all, but I was still mourning my father, and life felt fragmented. I was living a bittersweet moment, in love with my baby while wishing Daddy could have been here to hold her.

Beth had colic and cried incessantly, which exacerbated my postpartum depression and grief. I also suffered from severe headaches. My mother came to help me daily, reassuring me about the exigencies of having a baby. My body did not recover quickly, leaving me feeling anxious that something might be wrong with me.

Al was working long hours, and his absence from home left me lonely and scared. I feared failing as a mother, and I was exhausted. Breast-feeding was not fashionable at that time, and Al forbade me to consider it, so I did not even try to offer Beth my breast. It would have been more soothing for her had I been able to nuzzle her close to me, letting her breast feed. My low energy and uncertainty about motherhood did not help our baby with her reflux, and it was many months before she outgrew the condition.

We noticed cracks in our marriage as Beth continued to cry and demand my attention. In those days, men were providers and women were stay-at-home mothers. Today I see my son and my son-in-law fully vested in the day-to-day chores with their babies—changing diapers, feeding them, playing with them, bathing them. It just wasn't that way when I was raising my family, and it was common for the fathers to feel left out and usurped by a needy baby.

As Beth started to recognize people, there was a noticeable absence of bonding between her and Al. Beth only wanted me. This frustrated and upset Al, who on one occasion, in a misguided attempt to address the situation, resorted to pulling Beth away from me, only to result in a screaming baby who thereafter saw him as a threat. The intense attachment between Beth and me was difficult for Al, and he became resentful of her neediness.

We were living in a one-bedroom apartment in Bayonne, New Jersey, which I had furnished traditionally with the help of my mother. I was juggling looking after Beth and trying to keep a nice home for Al, so that when he came home there would be a hot meal on the table. He was working thirteen or fourteen hours a day. We were both exhausted and overwhelmed. Little did we realize that we hadn't even begun to understand what it was to be exhausted and overwhelmed.

I was soon pregnant again. This time, I was more experienced, a little wiser, and looking forward to being a mother of two. Al was over the moon that his family was growing so quickly, although he only managed to relax on Sundays. We would stay in our pajamas a little longer, bringing Beth and her toys into our bed for a lazy morning. In the afternoon, we'd have made plans with Al's parents and my mother. The grandparents were helpful, bringing over whatever we needed and often looking after Beth. Since our family was growing, we decided to move from our three room apartment to a home in Livingston, New Jersey.

Two and a half years after Beth's birth, my water broke a week later than the due date. After several hours of intense labor, I was taken to the delivery room, and I remember hearing a sense of urgency in the obstetrician's voice as he sternly shouted, "Push down hard on her stomach," Of course, I had no idea what was happening, but I later found out that my baby was in a breach position. After what seemed like an eternity, I was put to sleep and awakened several hours later to learn that I was a mother to another beautiful baby girl.

How wonderful! Beth would be a big sister. They would grow and share their lives, become best friends, confidants, cheerleaders, and most of all, share all of life's wonders and travails. Now all I wanted was to see and hold my most precious newborn, but why was the nurse being so evasive when I asked to hug her?

After several hours of pleading to see my baby, our pediatrician, who was also a longtime family friend, came to my room. He gently kissed and congratulated me. However, there was something in his face, something in his voice, something in his demeanor that was just not right. Perhaps my motherly intuition was kicking in and warning me of danger ahead. "Jane, sweetheart," he said, "I have come to tell you that your little girl has some unexpected issues. I have already spoken to Al and your brother Marc, and we are looking into it."

I turned to him with panic in my voice. "Issues? What do you mean?"

I felt his distress and anguish, but he painfully stated, "We are just not certain yet, but she has polydactyl digits on the sides of both hands beyond the pinkies." Dr. Perkel explained that she had extra fingers on both hands. In and of itself, it would not be a big deal, but the baby would have to be examined thoroughly to be certain there were no other abnormalities.

My sixth sense was telling me that by the way Dr. Perkel was nibbling at the inside of his lower lip and holding his hand over his panicky heart, he was hinting at a bigger deal awaiting. Tears started falling down my cheeks as I asked if my baby was in any pain. The doctor assured me that she was not in any discomfort. "A pediatric surgeon will be here tomorrow to remove the digits," he explained.

I stared silently, exhausted and unbelieving. How could this be? Was I dreaming? Was this really happening. "No! Wake up!" I heard myself silently shout.

In the early morning, the pediatrician and my brother Marc, who was doing a residency in pediatrics at Montefiore Medical Center in New York, came to my room. I will never forget the look on my brother's face and the color of his skin. He was pale and ashen, and I could see how pained he was for me. We have always been a very close family, and what impacts one of us is felt by all.

With my brother by his side, Dr. Perkel began to tell me that my baby had problems, but it had not been determined how severe. They explained that any one of these issues could be an anomaly, but put together, they were a sign of neurological abnormalities.

As soon as they left, the baby was finally brought to me. When they put her in my arms, as with any other mother and child, it was love at first sight. She was tiny, but to me, she was mighty and beautiful. Yes, I saw the extra digits on her small hands, which looked unsightly and alien. I cried for her, because I did not want her to have any pain, and I cried for me, because I was afraid.

At five pounds and fourteen ounces, our baby's tiny body had a disproportionately large head. Later, my mother and Al came to the bedside, peered down at the baby, and refused to see anything but a perfect cherub. We decided to name her Suzanne.

While we were still in the hospital, despite Al's objections, I tried to put Suzy on my breast. She was unable to latch, so we immediately switched to the bottle, afraid she was not getting enough nutrition. She would cry with hunger, take the nipple in her mouth, but lose it soon after. I always kept a bottle close by so that when she awoke, I could try to put some calories into her, but it was never enough, and she started to lose weight. She would fall asleep unsatiated and exhausted from the huge effort of sucking. Then she would wake up hungry, and the cycle would start again. The nurses would scuttle around the bassinet, looking in on her, comforting me, and encouraging me to keep trying to feed her.

Because our precious baby was jaundiced, Al and I left the hospital without her. She remained under the lights in the neonatal ward until her bilirubin count was low enough to allow us to pick her up. (Bilirubin is a yellow pigment, and high levels in the blood may indicate liver or bile duct problems.)

Once home, I had a baby nurse help me for a week. With her experience, she realized immediately that something was not right. As the weeks went by, Suzy was inconsolable, prone to bouts of hysteria, particularly between 4 and 8 p.m. I was young and naive, and I had not been exposed to babies with abnormalities. I would stare at my infant, minimizing what I knew to be the truth. Suzy was not normal. She was not taking in any nutrition. She weighed less than when she was born. We were on the verge of a feeding tube. My mother and mother-in-law hushed my thoughts, and Al accused me of being an alarmist.

At the end of a long working day, Al never walked into a calm house. I was always in my robe, trying to soothe a crying baby as well as managing my toddler, who had become ever needier as she heard her baby sister wailing. My mother was at home with us constantly, trying to help me with Beth, who wanted only me. I was very mindful of how much Beth needed my attention and at all times tried to have a child on each knee, but it was tough for

Beth to get the attention she craved amidst Suzy's screams. I was physically present but mentally absent with my dark thoughts about what could be wrong.

When Suzy was at around three months, the doctors became extremely concerned that she couldn't follow light. She was also silent. She made no sounds of babbling at all. Our pediatrician feared that she might be blind, and suggested we visit a pediatric neurologist, Dr. Arnold Gold.

Dr. Gold administered a test known as high-density diffuse optical tomography. He placed a flexible cap over the exterior of Suzy's head. Inside the cap, fiber optic cables acted as conduits to discover the intricacies of her brain mechanics. The dispersion of light spilled the secrets we didn't want to learn. When the light didn't pass through and instead seemed to bounce back, we were given the news we *never* expected to hear. Dr Gold concluded that there was pervasive brain damage.

I heard him say "brain damage," and I felt nauseous, unable to catch my breath. What were the implications for a baby with brain damage? Was he really talking about my baby? Despite the problems in the first months of her life, I did not expect anyone to give us *this* verdict. When I was standing there in those first horrifying moments, my spiritual lioness roared. I was not going to abandon my baby to her prognosis.

Suiting up for battle, I did not foresee how rocky the terrain would get, how cold winter would feel, or how fatigue would become my constant shadow. I knew that Suzy would not be going to any institution, as was being recommended. I knew that whatever potential there was for her life, we were going to realize it. I didn't know anything about the neuroplasticity of the brain. I didn't understand where we were going to find help, or how, but I knew we would not stop trying.

In those days, there were no personal computers. Accessing resources was laborious and inaccurate. I had a teaching degree, but not for children who had "issues." Where was I to begin?

I started with our pediatrician's office. Dr. Perkel had the compassion of Mahatma Gandhi and the force of a Roman gladiator. He helped chart the course, served as my psychologist, and wanted Suzy to thrive as much as we did. He met our challenges with us, throwing his weight in the ring when we felt small. Every prizefighter needs a trainer and a manager. Suzy was that fighter, I was the manager, and Dr. Perkel was the trainer.

I spent every minute making inquiries. We only had landlines so I would sit at home, dialing our phones and taking notes on whatever information I could glean. I had Beth on one knee, with a book in her hand, and Suzy bouncing on the other. Often the person on the other end would ask me to call back because they couldn't hear me over the racket of the two children. Beth had become very clingy, and Suzy was inconsolable almost all the time. I foolishly failed to realize that Beth, reacting to what was going on, was suffering from anxiety.

Meanwhile, the woman Al married left forever. I became strong, courageous, and resilient. I was determined to give Suzy every chance. As a young woman, I had struggled with my identity, feeling overshadowed by my accomplished brothers. When I roared into action, even my mother expressed surprise. She never realized that her sweet, gentle, and agreeable daughter could muster up this fighter spirit. I was resolved to protect and advocate for my family.

My new self-confidence confounded and confused Al, who, having married exhibit A, now got exhibit B. At the beginning of Suzy's life, Al would often argue with me: "But Jane, that is not what the doctor said. You are making a mountain out of a molehill. It's not that bad." In my frustration, I would retort, "Did we go to the same appointment, Al? Because if we did, you would be either deaf or in denial. We were clearly told that her brain is severely compromised, and she won't function normally."

Of course, this exchange of dialogue was not conducive to a loving marriage. I had to learn to tune out much of what Al said to me, only asking for his opinion when I felt he could be helpful. How hurtful this must have been for him.

Al came home from a long day at work one evening and said, "Jane, I can no longer argue with you about your decisions regarding Suzy. We can only have one captain, so go ahead and spearhead the work. I will try to give you what you need financially." I deeply admired Al for having taken this bold step and for being able to voice it. For someone who wanted to control every aspect, relinquishing the reins must have come at a great cost to him. Although we often disagreed, at the core was the well-being of Suzy. Al was able to express his pride in me to strangers, but he couldn't praise me directly. I wasn't looking for accolades from anyone, but it would have been helpful to our marriage to understand that he was not as resentful as I assumed.

One day, after exhaustive research, I heard about a program at Huntingdon Hospital in Flemington, New Jersey. An infant stimulation program for children with developmental issues, the classes consisted of activities that aroused or stimulated a baby's sense of sight, sound, touch, taste, and smell. The classes trained the baby's curiosity, attention span, memory, and nervous system development. We were encouraged to repeat the exercises repeatedly, as the amount of stimulation that the baby received directly affected how many synapses were formed.

The hospital was an hour and a half drive each way. We didn't have Google Maps in those days, so Al accompanied me to the first couple of appointments to make sure I didn't lose my way. My mother took charge of Beth, who had become so attached to me that she would wail whenever I left her alone. My mother-in-law helped with the shopping and babysat, even though she was skeptical of the doctor's reports and worried about her son.

Al was working horrendously long hours to build the business and our financial security. None of the medical treatment was covered by insurance, and Al took his responsibilities seriously.

Fall was beginning, and days were getting shorter. This meant that at 6.00 a.m., leaving the house for the lessons became colder and darker. I wended my way through the brown and orange leaves, and then through the ice and snow, to be prompt for the 8.00 a.m. start time.

We were a group of six babies and six moms. We trained together for two hours, four mornings a week. Parents were encouraged to be fully present at these sessions, mastering the exercises so that we could continue them at home. We bombarded their little brains with stimuli. I remember massaging Suzy's arms and legs, tickling her skin, and putting a light lavender smell in front of her nose.

The moms in the class became close confidants, and they were a great source of comfort to me. We swapped new information and hugged each other when one of the babies responded positively, giving us all encouragement and optimism. We all had a very special love for our little angels, but were racked with guilt that we couldn't protect them from the difficulties they would encounter in their lives. We were training for a marathon, each one promising to make it over the finish line, no matter how long it took.

Because Suzy's milestones were so delayed, each time she showed a little progress, I came home to regale the family with her new achievement. Her first smile was at five months. If you have been a parent, you will understand the significance of a baby's first social smile—an intentional gesture of loving recognition just for you.

The idea that Suzy might recognize me as her mom and respond to my overtures of love gave me so much hope. I hugged her therapist. "She is even more beautiful when she smiles," I said. "Thank you for helping to get her to this place." I rushed home to share her smiles with our family, who were always waiting and hoping for good news about Suzy. We stood in front of her day and night, making silly movements to elicit this smile for any reason we could.

When Suzy learned to laugh, she would laugh all the time. You could tickle her, and she would laugh. You could play peekaboo, and she would laugh. All babies are sweet and wonderful, but Suzy seemed to be sweeter and more wonderful. I've heard other parents over the years refer to their developmentally delayed children as "children of God." To know Suzy was to love her. She melted the hearts of anyone she met.

One of my worst decisions was sending Beth to a program at age two and a half. I needed to have extra time for Suzy, and I thought that Beth would do well in a supervised class with other kids. What a disservice I did to my child! She wasn't ready, and I still hear her begging me to stay in the classroom with her. Her separations from me were traumatic. Beth, darling, when you read these words one day, please forgive my stupidity and know that I was ignorant and desperately doing what I felt was appropriate at the time.

I felt very isolated in my struggle. I wanted to scream when my mother and parents-in-law would say there was nothing to worry about, that Suzy was just a little behind. Al was upbeat and continued to avoid the reality of the situation, which infuriated me. With or without support, Suzy and I had formed a solid bond already, and I was going to see to it that she got the help she needed to live the most normal life she could.

2

CLIMB EVERY MOUNTAIN

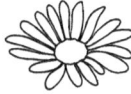

The infant stimulation program at Huntingdon Hospital ended when the babies turned one year old. By now, I had begun to learn my way around the world of special needs, and we followed the protocols to get Suzy into the Easter Seals program in Morris Plains, only a half hour from where I lived. Once Suzy qualified for the services, there were funds provided by the state to subsidize the early intervention program. We continued working on cognitive, social, emotional, communicative, and physical development.

To make the men feel a part of the Easter Seals program, one of the therapists organized a "Y chromosome rap group." The fathers were encouraged to bring in their gripes, their loneliness, and their fears around caring for a developmentally disabled child. Al was a trouper and went to these meetings with good intentions, coming away with increased awareness. After a reluctant beginning, he soon realized what we were up against. He was chagrined, sad, and resigned. After one session, he came home and said, "Jane, you have done a herculean job with Suzy. Please keep it up. Without you and your intervention, Suzy would not be where she is today." After that, Al would get annoyed with his parents and blast them for having their heads in the sand: "Can't you see, for God's sake, that she is not like every other child?" His transformation changed many things for me. I felt seen and heard for the first time.

We were a tight team at Easter Seals. The women became very close, the husbands formed bonds, and we went out socially, sharing triumphs and defeats.

Everyone had told us Suzy would never walk, and the staff agreed with the diagnosis. The head nurse and I agreed to try vigorous therapy to stimulate her legs. The first step was physical therapy to strengthen the undeveloped muscles. She was secured to a standing L-shaped board to encourage her to put weight on her legs. Her body was held in place with restraints. I was terrified seeing her strapped into this contraption. At first, she would be held up for two minutes, and then it increased to five minutes and then to ten minutes, each progression a cause for celebration and joy. Each successive increment of time meant that the treatment was effective.

When Suzy was distressed or tired, she would hold her arms out to me, imploring me to rescue her. When I wanted to reach out to Suzy, Mrs. Robinson, our therapist, would say to me, "Jane, if you really want to help your daughter, if you want her to walk, then learn to sit on your hands." I replied through sobs, "How can I watch her suffer when she is communicating her need for me? She needs me, Mrs. R."

She looked at my sympathetically and said, "She will always need you, Jane, but you have to learn tough love for me to get results here."

Sit on my hands and watch my baby tied to a board with white strands of nylon around her tiny frame? I hated this woman, who was asking Suzy and me to endure so much pain and suffering. I ran from the room so I wouldn't see those desperate little fingers reaching for my embrace.

With each day of therapy, Suzy was growing stronger. Her wasted muscles were starting to look more developed, and when at eighteen months, she sat for the first time, our cheers could be heard through every hallway. A major milestone!

Our next goal was to teach her to pull herself up on a chair or a table. Suzy was exhausted with the constant repositioning of her body to motivate these movements. At about this time, I started to notice how hard she tried to do what the therapists were asking. At this tender age, she was already showing her courage and fortitude. Although she cried for me sometimes, she also looked at me with a glare that said, "Don't pay attention to me until I succeed." I learned to let her struggle, giving her the space to figure it out for herself. It was arduous work for both of us. Most of all, we had to teach her independence.

Each day, we were there for four hours, and of course I stayed close the entire time. As if it wasn't enough to endure the exercises in the classroom, I then had to continue the exercises at home. We would drive home from the program, both Suzy and I worn out, but after a little lunch and a rest, we would start working on her strengthening exercises. I would hold her up under her arms, my back aching from bending over to hold her dead weight. She was like a rag doll. In warm weather we would do this outside, me pointing out the leaves and flowers in the garden to distract her from the task at hand.

Beth would watch us, gently giving Suzy encouragement. "Come on, Suzy, put one foot down and then the other." Beth walked beside us, smiling at Suzy with tenderness, learning how to be a big sister to a developmentally disabled child.

Mrs. Robinson was convinced she could get Suzy to walk but was not sure how. She believed in her and she believed in me, and I remember that her optimism carried me through many trying moments. She was a pro. When I met her, her strong handshake gave me confidence, and as the months stretched into years, I looked forward to her genuine delight at welcoming us each day. She never gave up on us or her belief that Suzy wanted to go beyond what the doctors had predicted for her. She recognized in my daughter the spirit of a fighter, and we both learned in those early years what many would come to recognize in Suzy over her lifetime: She would never give up. Even when she was in pain and exhausted, she pushed through till the end of a session. She motivated us every day to try harder. I felt that somehow, her two deceased great-grandmothers, for whom she was named—Sima and Sarah—were imbuing Suzy with their dynamic strength and power.

The psychologist at the program was instrumental in helping Al and me come to terms with our new life and with what it meant to be parents of a special-needs child. The statistics for married couples who stayed together, with this kind of stress, were not strong. With Jim's help, we navigated the way forward, although often fraught with tension and disagreement.

We were at Easter Seals until Suzy was three years old. Two of the other mothers, Carol and Vivian, became my best friends. They understood me, my situation, my personal pain, fear, and despair, as I watched my child, who tried so hard every day, to climb mountains of hardship. We shared a camaraderie that no one without a special-needs child could possibly understand. We were on call for one another at all times. We mothers were part of a club that we wished didn't exist. We were all depressed, all our marriages were in trouble, and we didn't have the luxury of sleeping in to recover from the day before.

One day towards the middle of her time at Easter Seals, Suzy was struggling through her therapies, and in her frustration, she threw herself on her belly. She had never done this before, and we watched to see how she would get out of this. We had been training her to crawl by placing her on her arms and knees, so we gave her a little assistance to remind her that this was how she was supposed to do it.

Someone called out to me from the back of the room: "Jane, did you park your car in the supervisor's spot today?" I turned my head away from Suzy for a minute to answer, "Not me." When I turned around, Suzy was mobile. She was moving her four limbs and making some distance over the rubberized mat. I sobbed, as did everyone else in the room. We were dedicated to one another, and when one child accomplished a new feat, everyone celebrated the victory. This was another enormous milestone.

When Suzy wanted to rest, she didn't know how to sit herself back down. She looked at us with an expression on her face that seemed to say, "Now what do I do?" So we helped her, showing her how to move her limbs back and forth and position herself into a seated position. When she was sitting again, she looked at me with a huge smile on her face. If she could have said something, it would have sounded like this: "I don't know what I did, Mom, but I know I did well, and I want you to be proud of me." I was a puddle. Other parents take these breakthroughs for granted. With Suzy, we were ecstatic.

Then something shook our world. We had become particularly friendly with Vivian and her husband Jeff, who lived not too far away from us. Al called me one afternoon as I was getting home with the two girls. "Jane, Jeff has confided in me that he is leaving Vivian for another woman. Their marriage had been breaking with the stress of their daughter's condition."

My heart dropped like a setting sun. Was Al transferring his own feelings and warning me of some impending catastrophe in our own lives? "Al, what are you saying?" I slurred. "Is this a hint of how you are feeling?" Of course I was aware of how much Al was missing his cute wife, but I was totally absorbed in my children and their needs and was unable to attend to his. I felt unattractive, unsexy, and messy.

Then in a soft voice, Al replied, "Jane, I will never abandon our family. I know I get angry and tell you often how dissatisfied I am with the state of our marriage, but you should rest easy, knowing that I will ride this through with you to the end." I have never forgotten how much his words meant to me that day. Al, when you read this, please forgive me for not telling you so at the time.

Vivian and Jeff's daughter Ali had been born with cerebral palsy. After the first year of living alone without her husband, Vivian could no longer find the strength to cope with the needs of her daughter as well as the rejection of her husband. She went into the garage with Ali and heartbreakingly committed suicide with carbon dioxide fumes in the car, killing herself and taking her daughter with her.

I remember the phone call I received telling me the news. Many ominous thoughts flew into my head. I was angry with Jeff but acknowledged that it wasn't uncommon under the circumstances. Why had Vivian felt so helpless in her struggle that she would end her life and the life of her daughter? Was this final act actually a sign of bravery to release them from the suffering that would surely follow them through life?

I thought I had been sympathetic to Vivian, so how did I miss the warning signs of her deep unhappiness? It's hard enough to take your own life, let alone that of your child. I can't contemplate the degree of pain she must have felt to take this final step. I miss her and hope that wherever they are, Ali is able to get out of her wheelchair and run on the grass.

When Suzy was two years old, Dr. Gold did a CAT scan of her brain. We took her over to his offices at New York's Columbia Presbyterian Hospital and listened to her screaming as they took her away from us. As a grown woman, I dreaded and hated the machine. How do you put a two-year-old into a claustrophobic tunnel and expect her to be calm? We waited outside the procedure room, horrified by the escalation of the screams. I can still hear them. Al held me back from marching into the room to rescue our daughter from the torturers. I vowed revenge on the forces of evil that were responsible.

After what seemed an eternity in my mind, but a half hour on the clock, the PA system rang through the hallways asking Dr. Arnold Gold to report immediately to the fifth-floor pediatric department. No one had alerted us, but we knew this concerned Suzy, whose shrieks were still blaring through the hospital corridors. Ten minutes later, Dr. Gold ran into the room, and almost immediately the noise stopped. We thought our daughter had died. I was on my feet, looking anxiously for someone to speak to. What had happened in that room?

Dr. Gold came out, came over to us, and said, "Do I have to do everything in this hospital? The damn fools couldn't find her veins to sedate her. I am sorry. It must have been traumatic for all of you. I can assure you she is fine now. I have administered a sedative through an IV, and we will report our findings to you as soon as possible." He stomped off, muttering something about sooner or later he would be cleaning the toilets to ensure they got properly done. I giggled nervously and yelled after him, "Thank you, Dr. Gold." He remained a wonderful doctor and friend to our family throughout his life.

The results of that CAT scan showed pervasive damage to the occipital lobe of Suzy's brain, which is the area that controls vision and focus. They gave her condition a name: ocular motor apraxia, or OMA. This is not a vision problem with the eyes but a neurological condition associated with the brain. The disorder causes problems with voluntary horizontal eye movement, so that the child is unable to move his or her eyes in a desired direction. The quick, simultaneous movement of both eyes in the same direction, known as *saccade*, was abnormal in Suzy's case. It explained why she was always turning her head in one direction or another. She was using a head thrust to compensate for the inability to initiate horizontal eye movements away from the straight-ahead gaze position. The vertical eye movements remained unaffected. OMA often leads to problems with balance and coordination as well as potential developmental delays. There was no cure or specific treatment available to treat the condition. We were merely advised to continue the occupational, physical, and speech therapy we were already engaged in.

Dr. Gold sent us to a pediatric ophthalmologist, who was intrigued with the condition. He had not seen many cases. When Dr. Baron needed to look into Suzy's eyes, he had to hold her head firmly between his assistant's two hands. As Columbia Presbyterian is a teaching hospital, many doctors were flooding into the room to look at Suzy. Interns, physicians, students, and specialists were all filing around the examination table to look into her eyes with cold, hard instruments. Al and I were furious as the doctors continued to force Suzy's head to remain still. Soon there were bruises under Suzy's eyes and on her cheeks, until Al and I could stand no more. Al boomed, "Take your hands off her. No one touches her again. Call Dr. Gold up here right away. This has to stop now."

Dr. Gold came up and took over. He said to the fifteen student doctors, "It's enough. You have confirmed the diagnosis. Suzy is not a lab rat. You have subjected this child to intolerable handling. Leave her alone!"

We still couldn't explain her inability to walk or talk. Al and I had undergone extensive genetic testing, but so far nothing had shown up. We were all mystified.

The work at Easter Seals continued. Fortunately, I was healthy and not prone to the colds and flu that were going around with the little children. Suzy, on the other hand, suffered ear infections, chest coughs, and other common viruses. If she was sick and couldn't go to the program, we did the exercises at home, so she never took a day off. I was a relentless taskmaster, encouraged by the impact of the treatments and their results.

Easter Seals held a class to integrate siblings into the world of the handicapped. Beth was about four years old at the time. After some playtime and a snack, the facilitator invited the siblings to share how they felt about having to share mom. "Do you ever want to see Mommy leave Suzy alone with Daddy so you can have her to yourself?"

Beth's answer was astonishing. "Why would I want my mother to leave Suzy at home? I play with her all the time." The psychologist facilitating the session told me he had never heard anyone answer this way. All the other siblings said they would love to have their moms to themselves. On the way home, Beth asked me, "Mommy, what's wrong with those children?"

It was the first time Beth recognized any difference between herself and those with special needs. She had just never seen Suzy as "one of those kids." It opened a door for me to explain to her about Suzy's handicaps.

"But Mommy, she isn't like those other kids. I don't see anything wrong with her."

"Well, Christina has braces on her legs because she can't walk, and Jill can't see; she is blind. Then Christopher has . . ." I went on talking about the other children in the class, and she kept arguing that her sister was perfectly all right. "Is she always going to go to school with those kids?"

It was an eye-opening moment for Beth, who eventually came to understand that her sister had special needs. It also allowed me to begin the conversation with Beth about the world of special needs children, and Suzy in particular. Although "different" her sister was a precious human being who depended upon all of us for guidance, support, and love.

Suzy always seemed to know what she was supposed to be doing, but her body wouldn't let her do it. At two and a half years old, she stopped crawling and refused to move that way any longer. She was watching everyone else, who was upright, and made us understand that she also wanted to be upright. We got her a device called a Rollator, which resembled an adult walker. She was moving around well on the Rollator until one day she stopped that too. I didn't know what was going on in her head. Perhaps she knew that other children were not using these to walk, and she didn't want to look different. We bought a panda bear on wheels and taught her to scoot around on it. With more strength in her legs as a result of the therapy, she would sit on the back of the panda, propelling herself along the floor back and forth at high speeds. Since the panda was now serving as her legs, we took it everywhere with us. This proved to be a huge mistake.

Al and I chose to pour all of our limited resources into our children. We were a young married couple with little in the way of assets or security, but we knew from the beginning where our priorities lay. We had decided very soon after the birth of our first child that we would go without for ourselves while ensuring the best opportunities for our kids. Nonetheless, once Suzy was born and we were paying for all her therapies ourselves, we found ourselves facing financial difficulties.

Al was exhausted. He would leave the house before the sun rose and come home after it had set. He was doing all he could to make his business more profitable. My days were exhausting—hours of driving and watching Suzy struggle with simple tasks while overcompensating with Beth, who needed attention.

Our living conditions were not comfortable. We had beds, and we had a table in the kitchen, with four chairs. One night, when we had taken the children to my brother's house in Pennsylvania, burglars broke into our house. We received a call from the police station: "Mrs. Fischer, I am so sorry to tell you, but you were broken into and entirely cleaned out of everything." Al and I burst out laughing, wondering how we would confess to the officer that the burglars had definitely left empty-handed, as there was nothing in the house to steal.

At this stage, Beth was a toddler, and my mother provided endless hours of babysitting. She would arrive every morning with the evening's dinner cooked and ready to be reheated. I remember coming home from a grueling day of therapies for Suzy. Al flopped onto a kitchen chair after a long day at work and said, "Let me guess what's for dinner! Macaroni and cheese? Spaghetti and meatballs?"

It was a little tedious, but with no time to shop or cook for ourselves, we were grateful. Without the support of our families, we would never have coped with the overwhelming demands on our time and money. It really does take a village to raise a child, especially one with special needs.

3

LEAN ON ME

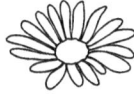

The Easter Seals program ended when Suzy turned three years old, so I had no choice but to put her into a school for developmentally disabled children—ECLC of New Jersey in the town of Convent Station. The federal government had not yet mandated preschool handicapped education at this point, so the Livingston, New Jersey, school board was not legally bound to fund children under the age of five. We were therefore responsible for a whopping $20,000 a year. Our appeal to the board of education fell on deaf ears since they had no legal responsibility to provide preschool services at that time. Al told me he would find a way to pay. He went to work earlier and stayed later. When it came to the education of the children, he was a stalwart.

The school was housed in an old building that originally served as a classroom for Saint Elizabeth University. Every morning I packed the two girls into the car to drive them to their schools. Arriving at ECLC, I carried Suzy up thirty steps to get to the door of the building. Once I made sure she was in her classroom, I rushed to get Beth to her school. I had a short window of time to do errands before picking Suzy up again at 11:30 a.m.

Suzy loved her classes at ECLC, and she was thriving. Her preschool teacher, Dawn Geanette, observed Suzy's incredible determination. Nothing was easy for her, but she met every challenge. The harder it was, the harder she tried. She gave 120 percent. Language was still challenging for her, and the few words she uttered were difficult to understand. Her motor skills were as yet underdeveloped. Because she would choke when eating food, I had to instruct her to chew everything slowly and carefully. I would deliberately show her my teeth, put a piece of chicken in between, and then slowly masticate the food, exaggerating every movement. Once I had turned the chicken piece into puree, I would lift my head and show her how to swallow so the food would not get stuck in her gullet. Although I had done the CPR course with the Red Cross, I didn't want to test myself in having to remove food from Suzy's windpipe.

One hot summer day shortly after her third birthday, the family decided to spend the afternoon at the local swim club. Of course, Panda came along. We parked him at the shallow end of the pool next to the rest of our belongings and went off to buy ice creams. When we returned, he was gone. We searched high and low, but he had been stolen. Suzy wailed that night and every day for the rest of the week from morning to night. We tried to replace Panda by buying every other similar item but never found one that Suzy did not refuse. Despite her limited communication, I understood enough to know that she would not let Panda be replaced. In our desperation, we placed an ad offering a reward to anyone with information that would help us find him. We received a few bogus leads, but nothing ever materialized. It was a horrible incident, not least because stealing something from a handicapped child is inconceivable, but also because Suzy now had no means of mobility.

The therapists at ECLC did everything they could to get Suzy to adapt to a new device. It was like asking her to use another set of legs. We couldn't believe that she was cognizant enough to differentiate one toy from another. There was just no fooling her. It was uncanny that she could be so stubborn and insistent upon what she wanted. This bullheadedness was the impetus for her to walk more quickly.

By the end of 1977, Suzy had become almost too heavy to carry around. She badly wanted to walk. I was still trekking up and down the street holding onto Suzy under her arms, urging her to stimulate the muscles in her legs. The neighbors watched us, waving hello. We marked the changes of the season during our daily outings by the layers of clothing we needed to put on. November, December, and January reached record lows, and the number of blizzard days reached record highs. Suzy didn't seem to care. With Panda gone, she had no independent way of getting herself around, and she developed a determination to become mobile. She wanted to practice all the time and gestured towards her warm parka and boots for the snowy conditions. I took her out on the cold days, bundled up and excited to put her feet down on the ground. Beth and Al would try to dissuade us from going out into the snow, but Suzy wouldn't hear of it.

Day after day, I pushed gently on one of her feet and then another, simulating the act of walking. When Suzy was asleep, I would fall into an Epsom salt bath and stretch out my body in the soothing hot water. The pain in my back sometimes caused my tears to drip into the bathtub. I was grateful when spring arrived and I stopped seeing my breath in front of my face.

Beth was an enormous help to me that spring. Although only in the first grade, she had such an understanding and love for Suzy. She was just a little mite herself but would come home from school and find Suzy holding out her arms to practice her walking. They would laugh with one another, fall down, pick themselves up, and start again. It was beautiful to see the love between them. Suzy was in awe of her big sister. Beth wanted Suzy to walk only a little less than Suzy did herself, and there existed some sisterly pact between them.

I had never weaned Suzy from the bottle or the pacifier. After a full day of therapies and preschool, I often gave her the bottle to calm her down and reward her for her hard work. At three and a half, I began giving her one bottle less every few days. Drinking from a cup was very difficult for Suzy because of her oral motor deficits. She could never coordinate sipping through a straw, as the lips, tongue, and muscles in the inner mouth were always very weak. Teaching her to use the sippy cup was quite a feat. Beth and I would show her the way every afternoon, but it was mostly unsuccessful.

It was the summer of 1978. Beth has just finished first grade. She was adapting to school and had made many friends. Suzy was approaching her fourth birthday. It was a boiling hot day in July. Suzy and I were walking up and down Blackstone Drive in front of our house.

I saw my neighbor Sam walking over towards us, and he called out to Suzy: "Suzy, Suzy, come to Uncle Sam." She walked out of my hands and took four steps toward him before falling into his arms. She turned around to look at me as she always did, this time with a look of elation I had never seen before. She was 100 percent aware of the momentous milestone she had just reached.

She wanted to share her joy with me, and I stopped breathing for a few seconds to let the achievement soak in. "Sam," I screamed, "Hold on to Suzy; I am going inside to get Al."

I ran into the house, calling, "Al, Al, where are you? You have to come outside and see this. Hurry up, Al." I rushed back to the street, where Suzy and Sam were having a moment of their own. Sam's wife, Lois, had joined him, having heard the squealing sounds of delight. Al was outside now. So were all the neighbors who had heard the commotion. Beth and her friend Lisa were screaming and cheering, and Beth told me this was the greatest gift she had ever received. There were cheers and tears all over the place. I thanked God for our miracle.

Every day Suzy would take one extra step. Of course, she would fall down all the time, and one of us would help her up, cajoling her to try again. She always had a bruise somewhere from bumping into a wall or a piece of furniture, but she was adamant about trying repeatedly. Over time, her balance improved. She grew steadier on her two feet, and her wobble turned into a gait.

I don't understand now why no one told us to do aqua therapy with Suzy. Perhaps it wasn't popular in the day, but it's obvious that floating in the water and learning to kick would have been the perfect leg-strengthening exercise. We had taken her swimming, but it was just to splash around a kiddie pool, not a therapeutic setting.

Having begun so many therapies at three months old, Suzy was habituated to them and never seemed to mind. Beth was attached to my hip as she watched me repeatedly working with Suzy. She would mimic me, and together we would recite the nursery rhymes with exaggerated cadence and physical movements. "Jack and Jill WENT UP THE HILL" (with our knees in the air) "to FETCH A PALE OF WATER" (we would lug a bucket filled with water). "Jack FELL DOWN" (and down I would go), "and Jill CAME TUMBLING AFTER" (and Beth would fall to the floor). We popped up and down, let our voices rise and fall, enunciating the words with clear pronunciations. If I was tickling Suzy's left arm, Beth was tickling her right arm. If I was singing and dancing, Beth was singing and dancing. She would pick up a doll and stand in front of Suzy, pointing out the eyes, the nose, the mouth, and so on. She was my assistant therapist and never seemed to mind.

I am grateful to Beth for her intuition not to treat Suzy differently. It is without question that Suzy's ability to talk stems directly from Beth, who chatted with her constantly, never minding that she didn't reply. When she began to babble words, Beth always understood what she was saying. Beth's friends never treated Suzy like a nuisance, because Beth never gave them the choice of exclusion. I can't remember now if she alerted her friends before they came over or if she simply expected them to figure out that if you wanted to be friends with Beth, then Suzy was part of a package deal. I do remember, though, always feeling that Beth was not getting her fair share of attention, and of course, later I was remorseful and full of pain for not recognizing some of Beth's anxieties as a child.

When Suzy turned five, her education became the financial responsibility of the Livingston school board. At this time, we were appointed a district child study team to assess her. Testing included psychological, educational, and social history. After the initial evaluation, she was classified as neurologically impaired, and it was agreed that Suzy required special services. The team wrote up an individualized education plan (IEP), which listed the goals and objectives for the following twelve months. I liked the team and trusted their evaluation. I may not have agreed with everything they suggested, but they were thorough and had the child's best interests at heart. Their doctrine of "the least restrictive environment" seemed to indicate that Suzy should go back to her district and start at a special needs program in the public school. She was progressing well at ECLC, and I felt moving her would be a mistake: "With all due respect, I am not taking her out of an environment where she has made such critical progress," I must have argued forcibly, because they finally agreed to pay for both school fees and transportation to ECLC. The bus collected Suzy at 7:50 a.m., and at 2:30 p.m. I picked her up for her private occupational therapy, speech therapy, and physical therapy, convinced that there was never enough.

Suzy was learning basic academics. She could identify numbers and letters, and although she couldn't speak yet, she was picking up vocabulary. The teaching staff was superb. She was meeting all her markers. Every holiday I went into the classroom with a gift for the teachers to show my appreciation. To teach disabled children, you have to be very committed, as the salaries are lower than in public schools and the conditions are demanding.

I had been talking to Al for some time about having a third child. He was dead against the idea, not least because he was terrified of having another child with problems but also because he saw the time commitment involved in raising Suzy. I had become consumed with the responsibilities of her care as well as worried sick about the financial obligations. Al couldn't fathom having a third dependent, considering what was going on in our home. I had always wanted three children and I desperately wanted Beth to have another sibling. One must remember that I had no idea of the genetic connection. We had been told that the etiology was unknown. It had been suggested that her issues were a result of the progesterone pills I took to bring on my period or the food poisoning I experienced during the third month of pregnancy. We were told there was no reason to believe this would happen again. Even Dr. Gold, the neurologist, couldn't give me a good reason why we shouldn't have a third child. The only negative was that Al didn't want one.

I implored Al to accompany me to Philadelphia, where my brother, a renowned geneticist, would facilitate a series of genetic tests on us. We included Beth and Suzy in the study. We had a round of interviews to determine whether we could remember any relatives with similar conditions on either side of the family. My father had one sister who was "slow," but out of ten brilliant children, what did that mean? Al had no recollection of anyone with a disability.

We underwent extensive blood tests, and when the results were returned to us a few weeks later, we went back to Philadelphia to confer with a panel of specialists. On a very hot summer day in 1979, the committee of neurologists, pediatricians, geneticists, and ophthalmologists told us we had no medical reason to believe there was any genetic connection to Suzy's condition. Therefore if we wanted to have a third, there was no reason not to.

Al and I began again to discuss the possibility of another baby. Many of his fears had been put to rest, and he understood my logic. Not only did I think three children completed a family, but I also looked forward to the future, wanting Beth to have support with Suzy's care when we were no longer alive.

I had a marvelous pregnancy with Ben, but he was a large baby, and I was in labor for twelve hours. I remember it was

Father's Day. The doctor was watching the fetal monitor and decided to do an emergency cesarean. Al looked over at him and asked, "You didn't think to do this before?" I was desperate to get the baby out and shouted at Al to be quiet: "Just let them do their job. Shut up."

When we got home from the hospital, I could not get control of my emotions. Al was thrilled that we had a baby boy. I was worried Suzy would feel displaced. Al had brought her to the hospital just after the birth. She would normally run to be with me, but she hung back next to Al, unsure of what this new creature meant to her. I couldn't imagine what was going through her mind, but I was very concerned. My mother and mother-in-law chipped in with extra attention to allay any feeling of insecurity.

The night of Ben's bris (circumcision), I was watching Al hold his baby. He turned around to the rabbi and declared. "I have my two beautiful daughters, and now I have my buddy." That is exactly what Ben became. He was Al's golden child. He met all of Al's expectations. He grew up knowing what his father needed and how to give it to him. He was always smoothing over arguments and placating his dad.

Beth, who was ten years old when Ben was born, was like another mother to him. Suzy, who always followed Beth's lead, eventually came around to see Ben as an adorable brother. As they got older, Beth became his protector, always coming to his aid if I ever tried to discipline him.

Because Suzy didn't understand how to interact naturally with a baby, her relationship with Ben at the beginning felt forced. We weren't able to teach her simple things like peekaboo or how to rock a baby. I got a life-size baby doll so I could teach her to mimic my actions. I sang, "Row, row, row your boat," but her sounds were more like, "Roh roh roh your boat." I showed her how to give Ben a bottle without suffocating him. She lacked the gentle nuances and calming movements that one instinctively makes with a baby.

The first year with Ben in the house was very difficult for Suzy. Ben gravitated toward Beth, who was more maternal towards him and loved him fiercely. A new set of problems arose when Ben started walking at a young age with greater stability than Suzy. Then he spoke with more fluency and better articulation. He was able to read at above grade level and became an excellent athlete.

When Ben was only three years old and I was busy running around to therapies with Suzy, Beth couldn't bear to leave him alone at home when she went off for her tennis lesson. So she whisked him off with her, and he became the ball boy for the tennis club.

At this stage, Ben started to pretend that he couldn't do certain things so that Suzy wouldn't feel threatened. We had to work very hard to make him understand that his sister would never have his abilities and that it was right for him to progress faster than she was because of her handicaps.

As the years passed, Al had done a phenomenal job of building up his business so that it was generating enough money for us to buy some furniture and put down carpeting. We were still not able to travel or buy luxury items, but our joy was never derived from material possessions. We had been able to provide for our family, and that was where our happiness lay.

Watching our brood grow in health and spirit, we thought about how our lives had been impacted upon finding out we had a special-needs daughter. I had read many books on how to cope, how to protect other children in the family, and how to live with the added stress of the situation. There was some solace to be derived from knowing we were not alone. I read about the struggles of other mothers and fathers in similar situations and tried to adapt some of their experiences to my own anguishing moments. But everyone has a different way of coping, and each of us faces different dynamics, so our life stories become unique to us.

I decided to approach our lives with patience and commitment. We knew we would not be like families with "normal" children. When my friends were planning charity luncheons with fashion shows, I was driving yet another hour and a half to a therapy session with Suzy. Although we tried to be part of a group of other young families at Beth's school, we bonded more with families encountering the same difficulties as ours. When we were in the company of parents with special-needs kids, there was no need to explain anything, no excuses we had to proffer, no behavior we had to apologize for. We shared a common understanding.

The most difficult item to manage was time. If I were a pane of glass, you could say I had been dropped and shattered. Each shard of glass sliced through the fragile fabric of my being, leaving behind trails of invisible blood. I was always needed and never available. I was always moving and never getting anywhere. I was a bundle of nerves, trying to soothe the frailties of all others around me, yet never attending to my own. My youth gave me energy, and my mission gave me strength. I remember very early on convincing my family to embrace the nuances in Suzy's development. From the very beginning, I recognized something in Suzy that I felt would be a guiding light for all who knew her. It was the way she fought for every milestone. It was her determination even as a baby to put herself through difficulties to learn something new. It was the way she looked at me and eventually smiled that reiterated her gentle kindness. Holding her, hugging her, you imbibed a force that transferred through her little body. This energy that she shared made you a better person.

Despite many hours of grief and desperation, we experienced many moments of joy and pride. Beth and Ben were adorable, well-behaved, kind children. Suzy existed as an imprecise angel in all our lives whose light shone brighter and in more directions than all others. Our family unit was tight and strong, with love overflowing. Our extended family offered far more support than I had expected, standing shoulder to shoulder with us. There was something about Suzy that encouraged you to want to be close to her, to safeguard her, yet at the same time to draw from the special aura that she emitted.

4

MOVIN' ON UP

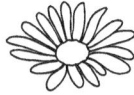

For two years, the board of education of Livingston, New Jersey, paid for Suzy to attend ECLC, but when she was seven years old, the ECLC principal came to talk to me. She said, "Suzy's strength is her sociability. Cognitively, she is on par with our students, but socially she is way ahead. I think it might be a good idea for her to go back to the district. She will be in a self-contained class with its own specialized program, yet she will be in a mainstream environment in the lunchroom, with better role models than she has here at ECLC." I had to believe that she was giving me sound advice, so I began to entertain the possibility of Harrison Public School.

The director of special education and the assistant director were eager for us to return to the district, and he agreed to put a codicil in her IEP that would allow her to return to ECLC if things didn't work out at Harrison. "Jane, since this is a pilot program, why don't you help us to set up the class?"

They were courting me, and I capitalized on the opportunity. I had already made my mark as a polite but outspoken agitator, but I was probably presumptuous to ask what the demographics of the class would look like. "You can join the teacher selection committee and propose a curriculum." the director said.

During the fifth interview, I knew we had found our teacher, a dynamic and seasoned professional who had all the right qualifications on her CV; moreover, she had the right personality. With all these accommodations made for us, we struck a deal to give Harrison a try.

Suzy was always malleable, so she didn't complain about changing schools yet again. In the beginning, I would sit in on the class, observing the teaching methods and the relationship between students, who were all at different levels of special needs. The parents in the grade had selected me to be the spokesperson for their children, and I felt the full weight of this responsibility. I would lie in bed at night and confide to Al that sometimes I wasn't sure whether I was an impostor.

I was extremely nervous about how the larger community would accept this pilot class. I thought back to one of my neighbors, who would rush past us while we were waiting for the bus in the morning, as if Suzy's condition were contagious.

Suzy was in the second grade when she started at Harrison. At least that was her chronological grade, but obviously she was not learning at a second-grade level. The eight children in her class were of varying levels of proficiency. Some were higher-functioning, some were lower, but Suzy remained the most socially adept. She was popular, and she would have occasional play dates after school.

But I was remiss in believing that the entire grade was friendly with Suzy. I had recently taken up the baton for inclusion and insisted that the children with special needs be part of the mainstream. I spent my days and nights arguing with school boards, attending meetings with superintendents, and listening to the advice of social workers and psychologists. I was now on the committee for children with special needs in Livingston and was a representative on the parent-teachers council.

Suzy's walking was stable, and her speech had become comprehensible to most people. She was meeting the goals in her individual educational program, which was reassessed on an annual basis in the spring. I wanted her to be introduced to a computer, but her child study team and the case manager felt it would be a waste of time. I was told, "Suzy cannot even write. Look at her IQ. She will never learn to use a keyboard. You are being completely unrealistic in what you think she will accomplish. If she ever learns to tie her shoe, it will be fortunate."

Al was outraged, and I was crazed. We hired an independent evaluator, Dr. Jack Goralsky, to test Suzy's capabilities. He presented his results at a meeting with the director of special education, the child study team, and the case manager. "You say you won't teach her the keyboard? Why would you not even attempt to help her with this skill? Yes, her motor scores are low, and she is deficient in tactile abilities, but that doesn't mean she isn't teachable. Nor does it mean that you don't try to introduce her to a new modality."

The meeting had become very contentious. I continued, exasperated: "Have you even been in to talk to Suzy? Are you just going to assume that at eight years old she is never going to be able to do anything with her life based on some test scores?" I was shaking with anger. "You have to revise the way you are thinking about her. Yes, she is disabled, but she needs to learn life skills. She must learn to dress herself. She doesn't need to learn about latitude and longitude, but she needs to know what state she lives in. She doesn't have to learn to read a map, but she has to know that the blue on the map represents water."

The director of special education was nodding in agreement; I had one ally in the room. The child study team was looking at me with daggers in their eyes.

I continued my tirade: "I am not going to accept that Suzy is incapable of learning to work on a keyboard. It is simply not true. Suzy is capable of learning many skills if the time is invested in teaching her." This day was a very big turning point in Suzy's educational life.

I was a tough opponent, but Al was tougher, and together we resisted the archaic standards of the educational world. I became entrenched in the system of special needs learning, although I still didn't have my master's degree. I started a PTA, Parents and Professionals for Exceptional Children, and I was appointed the first president of the group. I gained a reputation for polite perseverance, and I was called the "gentle barracuda."

Suzy graduated from Harrison at the end of the fourth grade. Most of the children from her class moved with her to the next school, which was Collins. The principal at Collins was very welcoming and eager to work alongside me. My involvement with the school system had grown, and at Collins, my crusade for inclusion became my gospel. I believed that every child had the God-given right to be included, and I brought that message along to every meeting. But as I learned later, it's also everyone's God-given right to choose where they would like to be included.

Suzy was still young and doing everything grown-ups suggested. She was a delightfully happy child, who got up for school every morning with a smile on her face and excited to learn her lessons. I never had to fight with her to be on time. I never had to cajole her to get on the bus.

Her classmates used to love coming over to our house after school. We always had fun activities for engaging them. Occasionally I would tell Suzy to invite a friend over for an afternoon of baking. We would put on aprons, and I would give the two of them flour and milk to mix. Then I would show them how to break an egg on the side of a bowl so that the shell did not fall into the yolk or the white. We'd mix up batches of cookie dough until there was flour all over the floor and the tables. After the cupcakes came out of the oven, I would give them sprinkles and icing with which to decorate.

I knew how much Suzy loved her social life, so when she wasn't doing extra therapies, I kept her busy with friends. I remember one little girl who was very high-functioning but extremely anxious and perhaps autistic. Years later, I found out that she actually got married and had children. We lost touch with her, but I hope she made a success of her family life.

There was a great difference between the friendships that Suzy had and the ones that Beth had. Beth's friends would sleep over. I could leave them alone in the basement or in her bedroom, confident that they wouldn't burn the house down. Suzy and her friends always had to be supervised.

Our house was filled with activity. On one occasion, the mother of one of Suzy's friends came to pick her child up, and he had somehow escaped from our supervision. I was panicked about where he might be and very embarrassed that the mother would think this was how we ran our home. We called for him several times, but he did not answer. As I was walking through the hallway, I noticed a bump behind the curtain. I walked over and there he was, hiding from his mother so she couldn't take him from our house. She went to get him, but he resisted saying, "No, Momma, I don't want to go home to our house. Suzy's house has better toys, and her mother bakes cupcakes with us."

That year, there was a spring assembly, and the fifth grade was selected to perform. The parents of the children in the self-contained classes were invited to join. What should have been a momentous occasion for the merits of inclusion turned into a debacle of segregation. Al and I were excited to watch the performance, but upon entering the auditorium, we were astounded to see Suzy and her classmates on the gym floor while the "normal" fourth graders were on the stage. Both groups were attempting to perform the same material, but only a blind man would have failed to see the separation between the two groups.

I was furious. Al had to hold me in my seat to prevent me from running to lift those children up and put them on the stage. I anguished through the assembly, irate at the callous ignorance of the administration that had made this decision.

Despite my fury, I applauded politely and commended the staff and children for a job well done. But when it was over, Al and I marched into the principal's office without an appointment. "How could you have allowed this decision?" we said. "What were you thinking? By separating and singling out our children with special needs, you have exacerbated the very issue I have tried to eradicate."

He was totally shocked by our reaction: "I included them, didn't I?"

I have tried to make excuses for him for thirty-five years. In his mind, just including the kids was enough. When I asked him why on earth he felt having them perform on the floor of the gym rather than the stage was acceptable, he replied, "In all sincerity, I thought they would be more comfortable."

I determined that it would be more beneficial for me to turn this into a teaching moment rather than a punitive one. I called for a meeting with the director of special services, all the staff, and the principal. We talked about what inclusion really meant. It certainly did not constitute a token appearance! Admittedly, we have come a long way since those early days of inclusion.

It was time for me to teach Suzy a valuable lesson. She had come home from school, asking why I was so upset. I told her that I was very proud of her performance, but I was troubled that her group was not on the stage. I explained that I had already spoken to her principal. She ever so sweetly urged me not to be upset: "Mom, don't be angry with him. He is a very nice man, and he meant well." I explained that sometimes meaning well is just not enough. We talked about how she had every right to be on the stage with the rest of her class and not be discriminated against. I believe it was a defining moment for many reasons.

Growing up in a Jewish home, Suzy was familiar with Shabbat dinners, the High Holy Days, the lighting of the candles, and other common Jewish traditions. Beth had been attending classes at the synagogue, and Suzy had expressed a curiosity for doing the same. Al and I, along with another family whose son had learning disabilities, approached the synagogue about starting a program in Jewish education for children with handicaps. The rabbi was very supportive and suggested that we prepare a curriculum package with goals and requirements for the board of education, which would need to rubber-stamp an additional class at the Hebrew school.

The proposal seemed to be universally accepted, except for one or two congregants who couldn't understand why "they" would need to attend Hebrew school, because what could "they" possibly get out of it? One particularly unpleasant human was overheard saying, "It's like cancer. You don't want it, but you don't have the choice to say no to it."

There had never been a program of this sort in the community, and we were besieged with requests. We were unsure what the results would be, but that wasn't the point of the program. There were seven children in the first class. Although they were a self-contained study class, they were incorporated into the larger group of students during the holidays, services, events, and activities.

We hired a competent teacher who inspired the children to learn, sing, dance, and recognize prayers. When teaching them about the biblical characters, she mentioned that Moses spoke with a lisp. Suzy was so excited coming home that day, exclaiming, "Mommy, Moses also has a speech problem. We have so much in common."

Most children didn't like going to Hebrew school, but Suzy loved it. Three days a week, she would be standing next to the door, ready in her jacket and boots to get into the carpool. Beth, now a teenager, was humiliated. "Mom, tell Suzy to get away from the front door. She is so uncool." Suzy did everything with zeal. She would show up to her class and ask her teacher what good deeds they could do that day. She loved offering services to others. It was hard to dampen her spirits.

5

You Can Fly

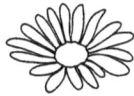

When Al and I went to visit sleepaway camps with our son, Ben, we took Suzy along with us. The camps were geared towards high-functioning individuals, but the staff was always solicitous and answered Suzy's questions as if she could one day attend. Suzy's enthusiasm has always been a catalyst to melt hearts, and the camp administration was no exception.

With each facility we visited, Suzy would become more and more insistent on her own attendance, and with her penchant for repetition badgered me relentlessly. How ironic that Beth, who was the ideal candidate, was reluctant to go, but it was all Suzy could think about.

I don't think Al thought it was a bad idea at all. It would certainly provide me with some respite, and he might have enjoyed some alone time with his wife. I was more reluctant to agree to this arrangement, because now Suzy and I had a mutually symbiotic relationship. I worried about her falling and getting hurt or not being able to master a skill, even one modified to her capabilities. I had never allowed her to be apart from me. She had never slept outside of the house.

"Suze," I said, "Let's talk about this more next year. You know I would miss you so much." As the words glided off my tongue, I reflected on my selfishness. Whom was I thinking about when I made that statement?

Al completed the decision-making. "I believe that we can talk Mom into letting you go," he told Suzy. "I'm going to sit with her and discuss all the pros and cons. I feel confident that she will agree to it." He used a tone that said, "You sit this one out. I'm taking over here." He was right.

Later that night, Al admonished me in an uncharacteristically gentle way: "Jane, you are winning the war and losing the battle. You have fought for years to enable Suzy to maximize her potential. And now you are reining in her success."

I had become so enmeshed in my daughter's life that personal boundaries were unclear. We shared an emotional level of feeling that I could not accept anyone else setting foot in. Sure, I got tired and overwhelmed, but this had become the reason I rose in the morning. When Suzy triumphed, I rejoiced. When Suzy failed, I despaired. Our dependent-codependent relationship, which started from a place of survival and need, had consumed us. I didn't want time off, didn't deserve to relax. My identity was completely wrapped up in my relationship with Suzy. Ours was an entwined relationship, from which Suzy sometimes seemed to need to pull away. My focus had turned entirely to Suzy's progress, and I ignored and suppressed my own requirements. I had an unhealthy need to feel worthy by being needed. I had become a rescuer. A fixer. Suzy was the infirm one, and I was the caretaker. She validated my existence in the world.

In typical Suzy fashion, the dog didn't let go of the bone. Every day for an entire summer, she nagged a little more. Suzy would ask me to read Ben's letters repeatedly. She would then sit at her desk and send me scribbly notes pretending that she was the one away at camp. When Ben excitedly wrote to us about shooting a blackberry (a slang term for an arrow that hits the black area of a target), Suzy begged me to buy her a child's bow and arrow set so she could practice in the garden. When Ben announced he had won the grand prize in the scavenger hunt, Suzy went around the house hiding various kitchen utensils, which we later had to find to prepare dinner. This wasn't easy, as Suzy was a devious hider.

Halfway through the summer we traveled up to visiting day at Ben's camp, with Suzy sitting impatiently in the back seat of the car. She was looking forward to seeing her brother, but more excited at spending a day on the lake and around the other campers. Having Suzy on a road trip of three or more hours can seem like an eternity, as she never stops chirping. We had brought favors for the boys in Ben's bunk, and Suzy wanted to distribute them.

We arrived a little early, and she tumbled out of the car and ran to find Ben's bunkhouse. "Hello, everyone, I am Ben's sister. I brought treats for everyone." Each bunk bed had been meticulously made up as if parents would be fooled into thinking their sons were always this neat. Suzy put a gift bag at the foot of each cot. The boys all said hello politely, either remembering her slightly from the day we dropped Ben at the bus or because Ben had mentioned to them about Suzy's developmental issues.

Other parents started coming in to see their boys, so we made our way down to the lake with Ben, carefully trying to make this day about him. Ben wanted to show us his water-skiing tricks, so we located a shady wooden bench under an

Eastern red cedar on the edge of the water. We watched as Ben hunkered in position in the water with the skis between his feet, as he had been instructed. Suzy was straining to see him, so she ran down to the edge of the lake, tripping over some small stones, and falling into the cool water. I knew she could tread water, so I didn't panic, but a couple of counselors dived into the water. She came out with someone on each side of her, a grin from ear to ear, and said, "Mom, that was nice and refreshing, but I hope you weren't worried about me. Can you please get me a towel?"

Of course, the incident drew our focus away from Ben. "Darling, I am so sorry we missed your waterskiing turn. Please tell us what you would like to do next." Although I believed that he needed my overcompensation, this was not at all Ben's character. He shook off my attention, instead going over to Suzy, he gave her a hug and said in his characteristically kind, understanding, and funny way, "Suz, life is never dull around you. You always keep us on our toes."

After an exhausting day of color wars, picnic lunch, and small talk with other families, we drove back into the city with our permanently pleasant, mentally challenged daughter. Suzy just wanted to be like everyone else and excitedly described the activities she enjoyed the most.

The next spring, I located a facility for special needs campers and put in an application. The camp director called us to politely decline our attendance: "Jane, I am so sorry to tell you this. I have read and reread the reports, and Suzy does not fit the level of camper that we can handle here."

I knew what her reports said; of course I knew. I had met this resistance many times before. "Jim," I replied, "please give me the opportunity to bring Suzy up to Utica to meet with you.

If you still feel this way after you spend some time with her, I promise not to bother you again." I used a tone that I had used innumerable times before. Confident and unemotional, as if I was talking about a student rather than my own daughter. The blustery reply was insipid: "I can't let you waste your money like that. It's an expensive trip, and I don't know if it will be worth your while."

"Listen, Jim, it's my money and my time, and I don't mind losing a little of either." With a reluctant mutter, Jim agreed, and we set a date.

The day of travel was wretched. The plane rocked and bucked, and as someone who has never enjoyed flying, I held on to my seat base in fear of being thrown about the plane. Suzy looked over at me and said, "Mommy, relax. Give me your hand." I suppose she had learned this reaction from the countless times I had given it to her.

Jim and his staff met us at the camp gates. Immediately Suzy lit up and told him how happy she was to be there. She smiled that sweet, sweet smile, and I felt his premature judgment tempering. Suzy was elated, overflowing with joy at each new discovery. She skipped across the huge grounds, going from one activity to another, sharing her huge enthusiasm to participate.

It was April, and there were quite a few counselors preparing the camp for the summer. "Hello," she said, "my name is Suzy Fischer, and I really want to come to this camp this summer." When she saw the archery instructor fiddling with the equipment, she asked her, "Are you the coach this summer? My brother has learned archery, and I want to learn as well." She toured the kitchen and told the chefs she ate everything except pork. She shrieked when she saw the slides tumbling into the lake. She retrieved eggs from the chickens, clucking while the goats nuzzled at her fingers. She had found a paradise, and she wasn't shy about sharing her feelings.

The director stayed next to us throughout the day, evaluating Suzy and looking at me with curiosity and confusion. I had never seen her this animated. It was not a show to ingratiate herself to the camp director. She bubbled over with her fearless affirmations: "Jim, this is so wonderful. I could be so happy here."

As our visit ended, I waited for his decision. Jim looked at me with a self-conscious gaze; his hand reached out to shake mine. "Jane, not only do we want Suzy here this summer, but I must apologize to you both for my original assessment. Her evaluations tell nothing about who she is. Promise me you will never let anyone, anywhere do what I just did, and that is to judge Suzy by report. Thank you for your persistence and requesting an in-person meeting."

I walked over to tell Suzy the news. She hugged him and said, "Thank you, Jim, I will be the best camper you ever had."

She was. She participated in every sport and hobby modified to her proficiencies. She was friendly, obedient, and congenial. She bandaged hurt campers, and she soothed the homesick. At the end of the first summer, Suzy was voted rookie of the year. For eight years, she traveled up to Utica each summer. She loved the creaky bunks, the damp, the insects, the starchy, unimaginative food. Although she was never able to waterski, she learned to aquaplane. They had socials, they had campfires, and she developed special bonds with the other campers. She became a role model, acting as an ambassador for new recruits.

Before coming to this camp, Northwood, Suzy had been attending a mainstream day camp close to home. She loved it. The owners loved her. But the campers just tolerated her. She was never included or made part of any group. Her best friends were the people who worked there, and once more, I missed the signs. Since Suzy never complained or told us she didn't feel as if she had friends, I ignorantly believed she was in a good place. Another blow to my crusade for "inclusion." I was insisting Suzy exist with "normal" kids instead of letting her thrive in her world.

6

HIGH HOPES

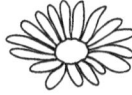

One of my biggest failures as far as Suzy is concerned was insisting that she stay in Mount Pleasant Middle School. To this day, I will think back to the years I fought for her right to stay there based on the campaign I was waging on behalf of the inclusion of handicapped people. The concept remains sound, but it is not a one-size-fits-all theory. I have given lectures about the need to make gradations and adjustments to suit the individual and the handicap. For example, those suffering from blindness or deafness always wish to be included, so there must be choices available for them. But in my daughter's case, I was egotistical and myopic.

Through my studies in teaching for the learning-disabled, I became a disciple of the renowned psychologist Professor Reuven Feuerstein. As a refugee to the new state of Israel along with many Holocaust survivors in 1948, he observed some of the surviving children who had developed behavior patterns that seemed to indicate they were "retarded" and "uneducable." Reuven, who was a deeply religious man, believed that all children have the spirit of the Divine within and, irrespective of their developmental problems, should be helped.

Feuerstein created a mediated learning experience (MLE), which encouraged assessors to adjust material to suit a particular child's difficulties. The premise was that a child with developmental disabilities, having to undergo the same standardized methods as the general population, would be limited in his or her ability to complete the tasks. Evaluators were taught to include singing, dancing, or rolling on the floor instead of sitting still at the testing table. Simply increasing the time allowed on the test helped with comprehension and cognition.

The brain's ability to change and adapt, called structural cognitive modifiability (SCM) theory, suggests that people can improve their thinking and problem-solving skills. To put this theory into practice, Feuerstein created two important tools.

The first tool, LPAD (learning potential assessment device), helps identify a person's ability to learn and grow rather than just measuring their intelligence. It focuses on what someone can do well and uses that as a starting point for teaching.

The second tool, IE (instrumental enrichment), consists of exercises on paper designed to boost thinking skills and overcome obstacles. It's useful for people facing challenges or looking to enhance their problem-solving abilities.

What's great about IE is that it not only helps improve cognitive skills but also boosts a student's confidence and attitude towards learning. Individuals could even use its problem-solving skills to learn to deal with everyday issues, like getting the trash collected or managing noise in their buildings.

In the winter of 1985, when Suzy was eleven years old and at Mount Pleasant, I was approached to let her participate in a study that Dr. Kevin Keane was conducting at Columbia University. I explained to Suzy what they were going to be looking for, and as usual she was happy to go along with it. As a practitioner of LPAD and IE, Dr. Keane was looking to illustrate that IQ scores are invalid for children with disabilities, and that by offering a mediated style of learning, he could successfully teach them how to accomplish tasks.

I asked Suzy's teacher, Laura, to accompany us. Laura never limited any child with her quote "you can do it" motto and her optimistic "no holds barred" attitude. A beloved teacher, she encouraged Suzy at every juncture.

The hall at the university was filled with 300 teachers, psychologists, professors, and observers. Suzy was cheerful and outgoing, eager to try what was being asked of her.

Kevin introduced Suzy to the audience and gave a little background about her: "Suzy has been medically diagnosed as neurologically impaired. Based on neurological examination, some hard signs of damage are evident. She also suffers from congenital ocular apraxia, although her adaptation to this physical disorder appears to be quite adequate. With regard to the assessment of Suzy's intellectual functioning based on standard measures, her overall score on the WISC-R (Wechsler Intelligence Scale for Children, Revised) dropped more than one standard deviation in the years between 1982 and 1985. Educationally, Suzy is currently placed in a self-contained special education class for neurologically impaired youngsters in her local school district."

Sitting with my mother, I translated the medical jargon with my own spin: "Basically, Mom, he is describing Suzy's failure on a standardized test that is given to all students. This is an unfair way to categorize her. It sets her up to fail. Let's see what Kevin achieves today."

It was a very long day, with many different problems set before Suzy. At times she was impulsive and looked to Laura and me for reassurance and approval. As the day went by, with Kevin's patient teaching methods, she became more confident and successful. His tone was reassuring: "OK, Suzy, let me show you how we are going to do that." He would give her a strategy to figure it out. "OK, Suzy. I want you to do this. The red is here. The blue is here. And now I want you to try to do it." Sometimes she needed a little more instruction, sometimes less, but after about ten to fifteen minutes, she would solve each problem.

In one exercise, Kevin presented a rather complicated drawing to her and asked her to replicate it by memory. This was very difficult, and she returned a scribble. "OK, Suzy, I want you to take your time; don't rush this. Tell me what you see." He took the image again and quietly reminded her of the extra lines and shapes that it contained. She tried again, and this time executed a drawing that had a few more defined lines but still lacked cohesion. They went back to the original drawing. He slowly explained what the illustration represented, pointing out how the various lines created images of a house, and she tried again. This time, she was able to reproduce something that very closely resembled the original drawing.

During the language portion of the test, Kevin asked, "How many legs does a dog have?" Suzy said, "Three," because she doesn't see the world the way we do. These are things that we learn incidentally, but her world is distorted. So he said to her, "Interesting. Three? Now let me ask you this, Suzy. Can you draw a picture of a dog?" Of course the drawing wasn't very good, but it had four legs.

Suzy never gave up. We were there from nine to four, with an hour for lunch. It was grueling. I was exhausted, and it was hard for her, but the harder it got, the more she persevered. Kevin kept looking at the audience and saying to her, "Suzy, do you want to stop?"

"No! I don't give up."

"OK, let's go!" said Kevin to the audience. When he asked, "Suzy, can you tell me what animal we get pork from?" She thought and thought, and then she said, "I don't eat pork. I'm kosher."

Kevin and the audience roared with laughter and appreciation. After all, do you give her a zero for that? Should she know that pork comes from pigs? Probably, but this is what he was trying to illustrate: many of these kids who are cognitively impaired don't pick up information from the environment, so to say they can't learn is not fair. They have to be taught differently.

At a quarter to four, he said, "Suzy, are you exhausted? Because I am."

"Well, I'm a little tired, but I can go on."

"You know what? I can't."

With that, everybody got to their feet for the loudest standing ovation you ever heard. They were whistling and cheering. I was riveted. I was crying. They were applauding not only her accomplishments but her will and desire. I was very excited, because this confirmed what I've always believed: that children with cognitive disabilities can learn if you give them the correct tools. IQ scores aren't valid for this population. These individuals, who we say are "mentally retarded," are "sentenced." That's not fair. There are many Suzys who are sitting in institutions and have not been given a chance to show what they can do.

In summary, Kevin spoke about her impulsive style, her uniqueness as an individual, and her work ethic. He also concluded that Suzy's manifest level of functioning is modifiable with focused, concerted efforts.

Having recently set up the organization PPEC—Parents and Professionals for Exceptional Children—I was pressing the subject of disability inclusion: including people with disabilities in everyday activities and encouraging them to have roles like their peers who do not have a disability. I was enmeshed in the political aspects of special education.

Suzy had been at Hebrew school since starting during fifth grade at Collins. During that time, we had given Beth a beautiful bat mitzvah celebration, and Suzy was now wondering why she was not going to have one. She always noticed what others were doing and never believed she couldn't do it as well. I hadn't thought about it previously, but I agreed with her: "Why not?"

I asked Rabbi Barry Friedman, Cantor Gerald Held, and her teacher what they thought. I stressed that it wasn't necessary for her to perform the same way that Beth had, but to do the maximum that she could do. Having gotten to know Suzy and perceiving her determination to learn, they unanimously agreed to begin the training.

Suzy had to learn the alliteration variation of the prayers, as she could not read Hebrew. The cantor worked one-on-one with her, teaching her to sing and keep a tune. He seemed to draw renewed energy from working with Suzy. When we drove into the synagogue driveway, he would wave to us from his window and then walk out to greet us. He took great pride in her achievements. Every night at 7:30 p.m. after a full day of school, after-school therapies, and homework, we would sit on her bed, listening to the recording that the cantor had made us and practicing the songs. It was extremely tiring, but Suzy wouldn't stop singing until she improved on the day before. She was learning more than we expected of her, so when it came to the day of her bat mitzvah, she could stand on the stage, full of confidence and dignity, knowing she had achieved nothing short of a miracle.

Aware that we would never be giving Suzy a wedding, we decided to make her bat mitzvah into a very grand ceremony. We invited 250 guests, who included friends, family, her doctors, and classmates. The invitation began with a quote from Robert Browning: "Ah, but a man's reach should exceed his grasp, or what's a heaven for?"

It was May 30, 1987. For the morning at synagogue, Suzy was dressed in a knee-length white lace dress with her hair pulled up in a white barrette. As she sat between the rabbi and the cantor on the bema, waiting to do her haftarah (passage of biblical reading), a huge shaft of light penetrated the glass dome of the sanctuary. It illuminated Suzy along in a glow of white radiance. There was an audible gasp, as all our guests noticed it. God seemed to be singling her out at that moment, bathing her with love and benevolence.

The cantor stood closely beside Suzy while she sang from her heart, the joy on her face singularly remarkable. We had been concerned she might get stage fright, but she seemed to flourish. My fear melted. The tears flowed, and there wasn't a dry eye in the house—particularly when she recited her speech and thanked those who had helped her, while claiming her achievement as a step to overcoming many more hurdles that she might face and declaring that she would try to achieve everything that had been declared beyond her reach.

It was a momentous occasion in the community, and the newspapers, including the *The Jewish Star* and *The Star-Ledger*, were there to cover it. The president of the synagogue was soaking in the accolades he was receiving on leading the first synagogue in the area to bat-mitzvah a child with disabilities. It would become quite a feather in their cap.

Suzy's theme that night was "Candy Land." The hall was decorated to the nines, with each table representing different candy collections. We hired a fantastic band, which had everyone dancing the entire night. At the start of the party, the MC asked everyone to take their seats as they welcomed the Fischer family. Al and I walked in first, followed by Beth and Ben. Everyone rose from their chairs as the MC uttered into the mike: "Ladies and gentlemen, put your hands together to welcome a very special, most exceptional young lady, who stunned us all this morning with her incredible performance on the bema. And here she is . . . SUZANNE FISCHER."

The applause thundered around my head as I turned to look at my beautiful daughter in a pink and white organza frock. She seemed to glide across with floor with a princess-like poise, smiling her widest smile, and evincing pure joy and pride as she listened to the guests sing, "If You Knew Suzy." What an evening we had! Suzy talked about it often for many years afterward.

Suzy's doctors had all expressed their amazement and disbelief, the neurologist, Dr. Gold, putting it succinctly: "Jane, she has defied the books I've written as well as read." He hugged me and added, "I don't know how she did it." This big, omnipotent doctor winked at me, insinuating that I was the wind beneath her wings. "Arnold, she did it through sheer determination, will, and grit. I just facilitated, but it has been all her tenacity."

Other children from Suzy's class celebrated their own bar and bat mitzvahs over the following few years, but four years later, the program had to close because of a lack of funds. I should have fought a little harder to keep it alive.

Suzy and Ben started taking tennis lessons at an indoor facility not far from our house in West Orange. Ben was a phenomenal tennis player and would watch Suzy, shouting encouragement at her. Joe, their instructor, was not a certified teacher for the handicapped. He was a great guy with a good heart who was prepared to modify the lessons to accommodate Suzy. He knew just where to hit the ball so she could return it. She loved the sport, and it was excellent therapy for her hand-eye coordination.

In 1988, Al and I started a new nonprofit, called Gateway to Social Opportunity. The mission statement indicated that we would offer Saturday socialization for youngsters with special needs of ages from five to twenty-one. The program ran from 1 p.m. to 4 p.m., offering arts and crafts classes, outings to sports events, meet and greet sessions, and some trips into New York to visit museums or see a Broadway show. For the first year, I ran the sessions together with a teacher, calling upon members of the community to volunteer. We were not eligible for funding from the state, so we were tuition-based, but we also did a tremendous amount of fundraising so we could provide scholarships. The program grew so quickly that we were required to hire more staff to handle the various age groups. As the organization approached its fifth year, I had to hand over the reins to someone else to supervise, as my mom was starting to decline, and I needed to look after her. Suzy looked forward to these Saturday sessions, when she knew she would meet her friends and do something interesting. It was a very successful program, and continued for many years.

Every time Suzy heard music, her body responded. Before she was able to walk, she would wiggle her torso and raise her arms in response to the beat. Once she was mobile, she almost preferred to dance her way around the house than walk. We usually had music going, since I realized that she was stimulating her muscles and getting exercise each time something was playing. It didn't matter if it was pop music, jazz, or even children's songs: she always moved her body to the sounds of the song. So I wasn't surprised when Suzy asked to go to dancing school with Beth.

I approached Doreen Kerner, who operated the dance studio, and she agreed to accept Suzy as a student, which was an incredible gesture on her part. We decided to place her with kids who were a year younger than she was, thereby making her difficulties less apparent.

Doreen introduced Suzy to the class as if she had the same skills as the rest of them. She always treated her with respect as well as graciousness, setting the example for the rest of the class. The other children didn't actually befriend Suzy, but Suzy was in a world of her own on the dance stage and didn't seem to care. She endeared herself to the pupils with her unfailing attempts to try every move, understand all the instructions, and look as graceful as possible.

The first year, Doreen suggested that Suzy be part of the year-end recital that the dance school put on for the parents. I was reluctant, afraid that she would appear to be uncoordinated and clumsy. Doreen allayed my concerns: "Jane, Suzy tries harder than any other student. I know that Beth gives her extra coaching at home and that she practices all the time. I see her determination in class. She is a part of the group and absolutely ready to appear in the recital."

We had dropped Suzy and Beth off just after lunch so they could prepare with the rest of the performers, get their makeup done, and put on their costumes. The girls were so excited, having run through their moves both the night before and that very morning. I was the stage-struck one. I hadn't slept, with the anxiety of worrying whether Suzy would cope.

We had met a few of the other parents over the year of carpool-
ing, and they were very understanding but a little condescending.
I perceived that often from strangers who didn't know Suzy well.
She would have been mortified to know that people felt sorry for
her or made exceptions for her. When being described to others,
she was called "the very nice girl with the mental and physical
handicaps." Why did people always have to be awkward around
her? Their embarrassment was not ill-intentioned, but they
seemed idiotic when they talked to us as if she didn't understand.
Once she overheard me grumbling to Al about an exchange with
a woman whose daughter was blond, blue-eyed, clever, dainty,
and would probably grow up to be a Phi Beta Kappa in a large
university with a first-division football team. Under the guise of
benevolence, she hissed at me: "It must be so hard for you, Jane,
and I salute your efforts to mainstream Suzy in extracurricular
activities. But all the same, it's not fair for the rest of the class if
they have to repeat exercises to accommodate Suzy."

I felt violent. I lurched forward with my fists balled, spit accumulating in my mouth and my teeth making a grinding clatter.
Fortunately, I saw the girls walking towards us and collected
myself. In the most liquid and honeyed voice, my tongue tripping
over the words, I replied: "How kind of you to acknowledge our
difficulties, Betty. I will explain to the other parents how you feel
and ask them to weigh in. If there is a consensus, I will remove
Suzy from the program."

Betty's mean-spirited comment and spiteful words were mol-
lified by discomfort as she thought about being called out to the
other parents. She countered with, "Uh, umm, no need to go that
far, Jane. I didn't mean that Suzy should leave the class. I was
just pointing out to you that she might be slowing down the rest
of them. But they are young, so it's not going to make that much

difference." I noted a victory for us as she backpeddled from her appalling comments.

Al, Ben, and I excitedly took our places in the audience. We had picked up our mothers and arrived early to bag the front-row seats where Suzy could see us and we would have a close-up of our special girl. I noticed Betty and her husband looking for their seats. I was going to point her out to Al but decided against it, remembering how angry he had been when I relayed the conversation to him. Why create a stir? I smarted thinking about Betty's brainlessness, but then the lights dimmed, and Doreen approached the stage to thank those that had assisted in the production. I could hear little whispers from behind the curtain of the stage and imagined Suzy lined up, ready for her entrance.

The older girls were going to open the performance, so I was on the lookout for Beth. When the curtain rose, there was a flurry of feet rushing to get into their positions on stage. Ah, there was Beth, gracefully appearing in the first line of girls. Doreen knew how hard Beth had worked to get Suzy ready for the show and wanted to acknowledge her efforts by selecting her as the lead. Beth was so talented, her lovely neck highlighted by her new hair-cut. Beautiful Beth, all grace and style. We applauded her loudly and called out a bravo as she executed her role perfectly.

After Beth left the stage, I saw Suzy following a line of danc-ers. She looked confident in her costume and makeup, playing her role with her consistently diligent approach. She moved through her routine with heart and soul, imbuing the specta-tors with profound appreciation for her efforts. After the show, Doreen proudly told Al and me, "She doesn't perform every step as taught, but she makes it look right. She was fantastic tonight."

To this day, I will think back with regret to the years I fought for Suzy's right to stay at Mount Pleasant Middle School. I was waging a campaign on behalf of the inclusion of handicapped people. I had not accounted for her peers' discriminatory prejudice and the stigmatization of "different" types of people. She was being tolerated, but not included in a way that she deserved to be. The school psychologist, Linda Halperin, Suzy's case manager, kept saying to me, "Jane, she is alone; she is always by herself." And I kept saying, "Well, Linda, if she is alone, then we must find a way to help her find friends. Maybe if we assign a buddy system, maybe if we go in and do some sensitivity training, we will educate the other children on how to socialize with people with disabilities."

"You can try it," Linda replied, "but you can't force people to include Suzy in a way that Suzy wants to be included."

On one occasion, Linda and I had an altercation. She was exasperated with me, my arguments, and my misguided determination. "Don't listen to me, Jane. Follow her, and spend a day shadowing her. Don't let her see you, though, as you know how she tries to please you. I can't convince you with what I know to be the facts, so go and figure them out for yourself."

I was chagrined with this dressing-down but cleared my calendar for the following Monday in order to do as she suggested. I perused Suzy's schedule for the day and figured out the most important times to watch the action: gym, lunch, and recess. I contacted the relevant teachers, and we worked out a plan so that I could spy on her but Suzy would not know I was there.

The following Monday I dropped Suzy off and pretended to drive away. I drove around the block as she walked into the school, came back, and left my car in the faculty parking lot. I stood outside the gymnastics class and peered through the glass inset into the gymnasium.

Suzy always did as she was told although one or two of the other kids were not listening at all. The teacher told them to warm up with a few laps around the perimeter. I could see Suzy trying to keep up with the pace of the group, but she sometimes struggled with the speed at which everyone else was able to do it. They split the class into smaller groups; each group went to a corner of the room, where they worked on a sport. Suzy's group started with basketball. Some of the kids in her group were on the team and wanted to practice their maneuvers. Suzy hung around, waiting for someone to throw the ball to her. Once in a while the coach would come by and remind the group to include Suzy in their play. The whistle sounded, and the groups rotated.

The next sport was gymnastics. The students were practicing on the balance bar. Suzy's balance is greatly affected by her eye condition and her weak limbs, and I could see her waiting for her turn with trepidation. Although the bar was very low, she had to lean on another child's shoulder to get on it, and then only managed to put one foot in front of the other before falling off.

Horrified, I waited for lunchtime. This time I stood outside the window in an open field. Suzy was in the middle of the lunch table. There were girls to the left and right of her. They were giggling, sharing lunches, hugging one another, and having fun. Suzy was alone. She was eating her food in isolation. She was trying to be brave, looking around for someone to pay her some attention. But no one did. Occasionally she would try to talk to some of the girls. Without being mean, they would answer her and then look away again, not interested in what she had to say.

Finally, I stood at the end of the hallway and watched her walk away from the lunchroom, completely ignored by everyone who passed her. I didn't even have to go to any more classes. What a fool I had been! My self-loathing frothed in my chest, the pain of what I had done matched only by the agony of my stupidity.

Later that day, I picked Suzy up from school, but this time with an awareness that I had stifled before. I saw one of the girls in her class pat her on the head with a "Hi, Suzy" and keep walking on towards her group of friends, and I saw Suzy looking at me and her eyes saying, "Thank God you are here." She could not stand the pressure to appear brave and resilient any longer. This is what Linda had seen and why she was nagging me to get Suzy out of that school.

This is when I cried. I went to Linda and said, "Let's set up an intake for ECLC."

"Don't beat yourself up, Jane," she replied. "Your instinct to try it was correct." But nothing she could have said then or now could repair the crack in my heart. When I think today of the trauma I put Suzy through, I would sooner lose a limb than knowingly expose her to the loneliness and isolation she felt.

On the first day back at ECLC, Suzy started down the stairs, then turned to look at me with pleading in her face. "Mommy, please let me come here. I could be a cheerleader. I could go to the key club. I could go to a prom." She was essentially saying, "I'll come to my world. I could be in my world. I could be part of the world." And she deserved that so much.

For me, it was defeat. I felt, "What didn't I do? What couldn't I do? What haven't I done?" At the heart of my soapbox stand was the issue of how inclusion affects the education of nonhandicapped students as well as how separation affects the education and socialization of physically handicapped and learning-disabled students. I've come to realize that although inclusion has become a popular concept and there have been many success stories, it isn't appropriate for everybody.

In Suzy's case, it didn't work. She was always tolerated but never accepted, and it was unfair to keep forcing the situation. As soon as she was allowed to return to her environment with others like her, she thrived. She immediately made many friends, and although there were thirty kids in her class, she was constantly considered the most popular girl in the school.

Suzy jumped into all the activities at ECLC, starting with the Key Club, an organization doing volunteer work for people in need. Whatever the group was working on, they initiated it, planned it, and then executed it—something that would not have been possible in a mainstream environment. One project centered on accumulating toys for the underprivileged at Christmastime. Another one collected coats and warm clothing for children and parents in the shelters. The group did a drive to give out eyeglasses to the homeless and the homebound elderly. The teacher often helped the club members draft a letter requesting the items they were working on that month. There was an opportunity to become a pen pal to a younger handicapped child, and although the handwriting wasn't always legible, it was a lovely way of mentoring youngsters.

One time, a teacher in a special needs class invited the members of the Key Club to talk to her students. Suzy spoke about how hard it had been for her to make friends in the public school environment and how she sometimes felt isolated but kept her head down and tried to concentrate on her work. She spoke about now being in a community with other special needs people, where she felt accepted and included and, more importantly, valued.

Suzy had always dreamed of being a cheerleader. Since ECLC had a program whereby students played sports against other schools for children with special needs, the cheerleading squad had many opportunities to perform at sporting events. After a number of rehearsals to learn the songs and dances, the cheerleaders were ready for their first performance. I helped Suzy dress in her uniform and went to watch her at the halftime show. My heart melted watching this group of eight young ladies jumping up and down, running through their dance routines with awkward movements, uncoordinated maneuvers, and unbridled enthusiasm. Whether it was at a basketball or baseball game, the cheerleaders always got enormous applause from the audience.

Suzy had a volunteer job working at Saint Barnabas Hospital in Livingston (today Cooperman Barnabas Medical Center). Her life was rich and filled with appropriate experiences. One year, she decided to run for treasurer of the student body. All the candidates had to speak in front of the entire school about why they should be the successful candidate. My brother and sister-in-law thought up a catchy slogan: "Vote for the honey with your money." Despite her inarticulation, her apraxia, her imbalances, and her cognitive impairment, Suzy got up and delivered a magnificent appeal for votes. She detailed and conveyed her strengths, including a sense of responsibility and honesty, which were important when dealing with money. She told the audience how much she cared, how she wanted to raise money for the school, and how many ideas she wanted to implement. She was a runaway success and went forward to carry out all the promises she had made.

Suzy has always been very social and loved the company of others. Perhaps because she has followed her older sister around for all those years, she became aware of the romantic relationship that might develop between a boy and a girl. During high school at ECLC, Suzy had a boyfriend. She mentioned her beau to me many times until one day when I was visiting with my aunt we saw a photo of him. They were dancing together. My aunt looked at the photo without judgment, simply remarking, "Suzy I didn't know that Gregory was a young black man."

"What are you talking about?" she replied. "What does that mean?"

"Well," my aunt replied sheepishly, "Gregory's skin is a different color to yours. His origins are African-American."

"Aunt Ann, I don't know what you mean. I don't understand." She had no idea of what Ann was referring to. Suzy was unaware of skin color. People were people. She did not distinguish.

Every year the school held an end-of-the-year dance, and in her final year, Suzy was elected prom queen, and this was the most special of all. Prom night was glorious. Beth and I had spent quite some time helping her to choose a dress. She couldn't decide between a full-length gown in a blue silk taffeta or a damask cocktail dress in silver. I was so excited for her that I let her buy both, so she could decide on the night which one she preferred. Of course, that decision meant buying two different pairs of shoes. Perhaps this indulgence was the start of the shopping addiction that has been reflected on my credit cards for many years. Suzy has been quite the shopper!

As the prom queen, Suzy wore a crown and opened the festivity with the first dance. She was very proud of herself, but the first thing she did was call all the other young women on the floor to dance with her. In her speech, she said, "Thank you for choosing me tonight, but in my opinion, you are all queens."

Suzy's date for the night was a young man named Paul. His parents drove him over to the house to collect her. We were all standing at the door when they pulled up. After a few clothing changes, Suzy opted to wear the gown with the blue shoes. Beth had gone with her to the hairdresser in the afternoon, and they had decided to blow-dry her hair straight, with a little curl under. The hairdresser had sprayed her hair with a lacquer to keep it looking good for the entire evening. I had helped her with a little makeup on her eyes, lips, and cheeks. She was radiant and exhilarated. She would have been able to go to prom at Mount Pleasant, but she would have stuck out like a sore thumb, and no one would have wanted to be her date, ask her to dance, or sit with her. But tonight, knowing that she was a star gave her the confidence and poise to walk into that hall with a gigantic smile on her face, aware of just how beautiful she looked and eager to show her moves on the dance floor.

Paul was a little shy and lacked any coordination. Suzy encouraged him to dance with her: "Come on, Paul. Come up and dance."

"I don't dance," he replied glumly.

"I'll dance for both of us!" she enthusiastically replied, pulling him to his feet. He didn't object, but he didn't move either.

Paul's suit was a little large for him and drowned his frame so that he seemed smaller than he was. He stood there like a stone, watching her as she danced for both of them. But he didn't sit back down, and he didn't object to her holding his hand as she tried to encourage a little movement from him. He began to sway a little, and as he relaxed his body under her zealous tutelage, a smile broke on his face. His parents and I were watching from the food table, and his mother burrowed her head into my neck, sobbing. "Oh, my God. What she just did was what years and years of therapy never did."

Suzy had participated in the Tournament of Champions since she was ten years old. It was an organization much like the

Special Olympics. Her sports were the long jump and track. The group would meet once a week for seven months of the year to prepare for the annual national competition. Suzy loved competing, and she did very well, sometimes winning medals.

As Ben got older, he became a fearsome athlete, and he took over Suzy's coaching schedule. Ben was ten years old and Suzy chronologically seventeen. He helped her embrace her abilities as she fought her disabilities, giving her the confidence to believe in herself.

They set up our driveway as a training ground. Ben would stand with a stopwatch and time her as she did her warmup laps. He had a whistle around his neck and the demeanor of a real-time coach. He put marks on the driveway and asked Suzy to jump from point A to point B. When she managed that, he increased the marks. Suzy never had a lot of stamina, so Ben would challenge her: "Suze, I am giving you thirty seconds to run to that tree. When I blow the whistle, you start." She loved her little brother in this role. They would both laugh and laugh, as Ben would act tough "Let's go—no mercy." She would say "I can't do it," and he would reply, "I don't want to hear that from you. If you don't do it, I am giving you double trouble."

On the day of her final tournament competition, Ben had a very important baseball game. He was torn between playing for his team or helping Suzy. Al explained to him that as much as he wanted to help his sister, it was important not to let the team down. Suzy and I were disappointed but supportive. "It's OK, Suzy, just pretend that I am there. Imagine my presence."

Suzy stood at the start of her race and said, "Mommy, I can feel Bennie standing here telling me what to do." With that, she went on to win.

As a side note, ECLC is still there. It is available to young adults to the age of twenty-one. They recently started a post-twenty-one program called PRIDE. Suzy was never a part of this, as she went on to another school, Maplebrook, after graduation at age seventeen.

7

THIS IS ME

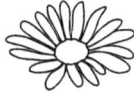

Suzy has always observed what other people are doing with their lives. Knowing that most of it was out of her reach always saddened her and saddened me.

Visiting Beth at college was a pivotal moment in the family. It was a winter morning in late January, and Beth was in her sophomore year at the University of Hartford. Beth had sent me a shopping list, which Suzy and I had gone off to fill together. On the list was a weighted blanket, which Suzy found confusing. I explained that a heavier cover is less likely to fall off the single beds. Then there was the remote-controlled outlet that Beth needed so she didn't have to get up on freezing nights to turn switches off. Suzy had always learned from Beth and was impressed with this gadget. She constantly emulated her older sister, of whom she was so proud and to whom she was devoted.

At sixteen, Suzy had matured to the most likely extent that she would ever attain. She was doing extremely well at ECLC, and we couldn't have imagined anything changing from the current status quo.

Ben, Suzy, Al, and I bundled up and piled into the car to take the drive up for Parents' Weekend. The bare trees bent in the icy wind as we approached Route 84. Typical for this time of the year, the temperatures had dropped to arctic lows as we carefully maneuvered the car over icy asphalt.

Since all the students were wearing heavy parkas and beanies, it took us a few minutes to pick Beth out from the crowd. We scooped her up and drove into town to meet her roommate, Stacey, together with Stacey's family for a bagel breakfast. Stacey was a delightful girl, and we had become very friendly with her parents. We arranged ourselves at the table, ordered an assortment of bagels, smoked salmon, dips, juices, and coffees, and noisily exchanged news since we had last seen one another.

The conversation turned to Stacey's sister Jamie, who was eagerly anticipating her junior year at the University of Delaware. "What are you going to major in?" "Do you know who your roommate is going to be?" We babbled away, asking all the typical questions one might ask of a high-school senior. I had noticed that Suzy was uncharacteristically quiet but didn't consider that there might be a problem.

When I turned around to offer her a glass of orange juice, I saw tears running down her face. "Suzy, what is it? Are you OK?" I exclaimed, surprised to see her so upset. I thought someone might have said something that hurt her feelings, but at that moment, she started to wail: "Mommy, I am sad. I am so sad, so sad."

I didn't know what had happened. I had never seen Suzy breaking down with such inconsolable emotions. Ben and Beth rushed over to hug her while a silence descended over the table. They both held her in their arms, also shocked, as Suzy was always so happy-go-lucky. With a cracking high-pitched voice and intermittent sobs, she continued. "Mommy, it's just not fair.

I am always celebrating everyone else's joy. I want to go away to college too. I also want a life away from my family."

We all stared at her, no one knowing how to answer this. I blustered through with accolades about how well she was doing at ECLC, and how proud of her we all were of her success there.

Then she said, "Mommy, isn't it time for me to have a little luck?" She was pleading with the universe to give her a little good fortune. Suzy's IQ silently trapped her in bondage, but her EQ gave her wings to want to explore the world. She realized that there was another way to live her life, and she wanted it. "Suzy, we will look into the possibilities when we go back to Livingston." I proffered, not entirely believing that I knew where to begin or that I endorsed the move.

On top of this, I felt terrible for Beth. What should have been a very happy day, all about her time in her college, had been usurped by the knowledge that Suzy was quietly agonizing over her deficiencies. None of us were able to shake off the morose cloud that had settled over that breakfast outburst, and we all donned a fake demeanor, replete with smiles and cooing noises, offering lots of "Oh, Beth, that is amazing." We drove back to the dorm silently, lost in our individual patterns of coping. I engaged in my usual overprotectiveness with Suzy, but also wanted to ensure that Beth was not carrying resentment.

When we had left, I had leaned into my hug with Beth and told her I would come up to visit again in a few weeks on my own, assuring her it would be a day for the two of us to share solo and spend it the way she chose. I hopefully left her with an understanding of my dismay at how things had unfolded.

I waved goodbye to Beth with a sagging heart, wondering how I could protect my family better than I seemed to be doing. I was feeling fragile, incompetent, and overwhelmed. I had never meditated before, but thought perhaps I might find some solace in a daily practice of mantras and centering. I had long ago ignored any warning signs regarding my own mental well-being, which was typical of what we did in our house. You loved and you fought, and nothing much in between. Someone was always angry, and someone else was always angrier. The tangents were unreasonably hurtful, and the resulting acrimony was left to fester into bitterness. This wheel of conflict perpetuated itself over and over, often rolling out of control and into a deep ravine with unassailable sides. Peaceful settlements were rarely reached, and our family had settled into their customary responses to oppositional feelings.

When the state classifies a young person as neurologically challenged, they are required to have a child study team of educational specialists assigned to their case. This team includes a social worker, a psychologist, and a learning specialist. For decisions regarding school placement, the team is called in to weigh in their opinions and give advice.

Our team was formidable, and my relationship with the psychologist, Linda Halperin, had morphed into a close friendship. When I told her about Suzy's wishes, she was very positive. "Jane, most children like Suzy never want to leave their parents. They have no self-confidence. This is a remarkable move that Suzy would like to make. I validate it wholeheartedly and encourage you to start identifying a suitable place. I will help you."

I was disappointed to hear her endorsement. I wanted her to say that she would not advocate for it. Why did she think it was a good idea for Suzy to move out of her home? We had previously believed Suzy would stay at ECLC until she was twenty-one years old, after which she would go into the prevocational program.

Linda continued speaking in an authoritative tone of voice: "Furthermore, Jane, it is what both of you need—a little distance from one another, a little separation. This is a chance for Suzy to try new things, to live with others who are like her."

Of course she was correct. My trepidation was driven by my own emotional needs. Suzy had been away to camp for seven weeks, and those were the best summers of her life. She would return at the end of the session with joy, having learned new skills and gained a new set of friends who were all looking forward to seeing one another the following summer. But that was for seven weeks. Here we were talking about the entire year away from family, from me. I was afraid of what I would do without looking after Suzy every day. I was afraid of her feeling homesick and missing the family—more specifically, missing me. I knew I was being selfish, but it was motivated by an overprotective zeal.

Yet Suzy wanted and needed this change. With uncanny emotional maturity that is usually not attributed to a person with her capabilities, she was insisting that we both get on with our independent lives. She may also have been offering me the chance to spend more time being a wife to Al as well as a more involved mother to Beth and Ben.

When Suzy had something in her mind, she would not stop addressing it. "Mommy, have you thought about it? Will you please let me go? Have you found any places?" Al was encouraging of the move and helped me with my research. In those days, schools had to send you brochures, and each time one would arrive, we would sit around the dinner table discussing its merits.

We weren't finding anything that struck a chord. That is, until we found Maplebrook, located in Amenia, New York, just on the border of Massachusetts. The beautiful engraved filigree gates opened into a campus that looked just like one of the finest East

Coast universities. The school was founded by three visionary women who believed strongly in the need for a boarding facility for neurologically challenged students. At Maplebrook, students had the opportunity to progress at their own pace and ability, so the range of challenges was very broad. Suzy could continue her academic courses while furthering her life skills and vocational work. There were plenty of sports to choose from, and socialization was strongly encouraged. Since the school was accredited by New York state as a high school and postsecondary program, she was eligible for tuition assistance from the Livingston board of education. Suzy had to qualify for placement, as with any university program, so we began putting together her test results and records. Just like everyone else who read her scores, the school administration was reluctant to accept her without meeting her. I assured them they were under no obligation, but I would bring Suzy for an interview, and they could make up their minds after that.

Suzy was ecstatic as we made our plans to visit. Determined to keep her expectations at bay, I said, "Suze, you know they must feel you are the right fit for them. They don't just take everyone they meet. So if they come back and say no to you, we will find other places. You must promise me not to be discouraged."

Suzy wasn't listening to me at all. She was daydreaming about being a college student and rattling off a list of dorm room decor items that she would be needing.

We arrived at the school, and Suzy immediately shook hands with the director, saying, "Hello, my name is Suzy Fischer, and I would like to be a student at your school. Can you please show me around now so I can see where I will be staying, where I will be studying, and the clubs that I can choose from?"

I took in the director's astonishment as well as that of his assistant standing alongside him. Later they told me they made their decision from that first greeting. Suzy has always had incredible social skills, and while she may have lacked in other areas, she won you over with her charisma.

We spent the day at the school, touring the dormitories, the stables, the vast grounds, and the classrooms. We got an overview of what an average day would look like, what the goals were, and what they would hope to achieve during her time there. Suzy hung on to every word that anyone said, gushing with enthusiasm and positivity. We drove back to New Jersey intoxicated with possibilities. We were over the moon with excitement, which we had to contain while waiting for various approvals.

Once back in New Jersey, we had to schedule a meeting with the child study team to request a change of placement to Maplebrook. The Livingston board of education was paying for Suzy's education at ECLC, and we had to confirm that they would continue to pay the Maplebrook tuition, which was more expensive. Since they would not be providing transportation, they would be saving approximately $20,000 per year. Al and I agreed to cover the cost of the residential program once the placement was agreed to. We received a guarantee from them to fund Suzy's education until she turned twenty-one years of age. When Suzy was accepted by the Maplebrook school administration shortly thereafter, we were able to toast the remarkable young lady, who at the age of seventeen was on her way to living her dream.

The week leading up to Suzy's move to Amenia was filled with dinners and parties. My two brothers and their wives, as well as their children, filed into our house for celebrations. The neighbors, our friends, and some of Suzy's classmates from ECLC stopped by with warm wishes and small gifts for her to take up to school. Everyone whom she had touched in her life wanted to wish her well.

When we eventually left to set her up, she was overflowing with emotions of self-love and self-confidence. As our car pulled out of the driveway, I felt as if we were in a bridal limousine, with "Just Married" cans dangling off the back bumper. Our entire street was lined with a sendoff committee holding signs saying, "Good luck, Suzy." My heart was full, and I knew that Suzy was crying tears of happiness and feeling all the joy she had been longing for.

I, meanwhile, was bereft. I needed to seek advice on my separation anxiety. I had just assumed that Suzy was going to live with us forever, and I had adjusted my life accordingly. Rather than celebrating her incredible independence, I was commiserating with myself on my anticipated emptiness. What was wrong with me? I had a career, two more fantastic kids, a supportive husband, a loving extended family, and yet I was shrouded in darkness. What was I without Suzy?

The drive to Maplebrook that summer of her seventeenth year was an amalgam of excitement, anticipation, caution, but most of all pride. I kept reminding Suzy she could change her mind and she kept shouting me down with, "Mom, this is what I want. I am sorry you are going to be sad, but you are going to be fine. And you need a life."

Despite my misgivings, I looked at my girl in the back seat with much love and admiration. Suzy had defied the odds once more and was now on her way to an experience that she viewed as a milestone in her development. She had worked tirelessly to get to this point. She never gave up. I remembered many times when the professionals had said, "Suzy that's enough for today." They would look over at me and say, "This is very hard for her, and she must be very tired, so why don't you take her home to rest now?"

Suzy would have her head down, never ceasing to pursue the task. She would ask for a few more minutes, and then a few more after that. She would not stop until she had mastered whatever was being asked of her. She had shamed many who wanted to give up on her: after persevering, she would inevitably solve the problem and look up with an eager smile on her face, saying, "I knew that if I had a little more time, I would get it right."

How many hours of painful therapy and muscle-twisting exercises she had endured to get some strength into her limbs? I remembered the times she looked at me with fatigue-clouded eyes, both begging me to remove her and at the same time imploring me to encourage her onwards.

Yes, Suzy had confounded medical science. But not without her own determination, hard work, and perseverance. She was the poster child for all things possible. She was a leader in her world, a kind and compassionate soul, who deserved more than she had been dealt.

Perhaps this was why I needed her so close to me. She constantly reminded me to be a better version of myself. Her love lifted me higher (just like in the song), while her need for me gave me self-esteem. Having a child with special needs infused me with patience and growth. I witnessed many miracles that soothed my soul.

Suzy and I had done the shopping for her dorm room. I wanted to buy excessive quantities of everything, while Suzy remained minimal. "Mom, it's enough. I am the one who is living here, not you. I don't need all this stuff. You must stop." She never liked anything excessive. I think it unnerved her to be responsible for too many items, while I wanted to make sure she would want for nothing. My other kids accused me of smothering love, and overindulgent shopping was a branch of that. On the way out, I noticed her looking at a jacket and incorrigibly offered to buy it for her. She retorted, "Mom, I was only admiring it as I thought I might buy it for you."

Setting up her room, we observed students with all types of neurological disorders. No two were the same. Suzy seemed to us to have the best personality, but we were biased, weren't we? She was bubbling over with hyperboles. "Mommy, isn't my view from my dorm room just the best view you have ever seen? Daddy, I think this is the happiest I have been in my whole entire life." And after an inauspicious picnic lunch, "Bennie, wasn't lunch the most delicious meal you ever had?"

Faking a smile, I winced each time she uttered these ardent exclamations of delight. What devil's vise had gripped me? I could not differentiate between my needs and Suzy's happiness. When it was time to say goodbye, my inconsolable despair dropped its guard in a puddle of tears. I cried louder and longer than I should have until Suzy hushed me and dismissed me with the words, "It's going to be fine, Mommy. You are going to be all right. You have Daddy and Ben at home, Beth not far away, and me just here. We all love you so much. Please don't cry." I was ashamed. But I continued to cry all the way home.

I had to become used to a very different cadence in my life, but I soon realized that it was a wonderful transition for everyone. I focused on my teaching. Al and I went into the city more often to see a Broadway show or eat at a new restaurant. I resurrected friendships that had been neglected, and I even went to an aerobics class. I took better care of my hair and my nails and bought some new snazzy outfits for our evenings out. I was finding little pieces of humor within my somber demeanor, and maybe even having fun.

Suzy and I would speak only when the school allowed her to call home, and I waited for these occasions like a castaway for a ship. Her words echoed with delight, tumbling from her tongue faster than she was able to enunciate the words. She never spoke of longing for her home or us or, more specifically, me.

Hearing her happy sounds, I responded with the cheeriest affirmations I could muster. The good angel on my right shoulder said "Job well done, Jane. You have successfully raised an independent and courageous young lady." The bad angel on my left shoulder said in a louder voice, "You are half of a whole without Suzy."

I had to live like that for a few months until Al and I went to the first visiting day.

My first glimpse of Suzy was brimful with dismay at her appearance. She had never been one to care much about clothes, nor did she have any color sense, but here, without my supervision, she was wearing badly mismatched clothes, which could have been cleaner. Her hair appeared not to have been combed for quite some time, and her teeth were not getting the same scrutiny they would have received at home. She was a little fuller in the bottom, and the socks were not a matching pair.

My prejudices melted the minute Suzy hugged me. I held her in my arms, and she whispered in my ear, "Mom, I am so happy to see you, but it doesn't compare to how happy I feel here at Maplebrook."

I backed away from her, stunned by her brutal honesty. I allowed my gaze to fall softly on her face, my eyes burrowing into hers. Although our hearts would always continue to beat as one, I told my egocentric neediness to temporarily stand back and allow my beautiful daughter to live the life she wanted.

We met her roommate, Joan, who, in contrast to Suzy, had been prepared early for a transition to a residential facility by a mother who lacked my support team. In fact, it was her dad who had primary care of her, and she seemed a little timid. Suzy immediately picked up on her mood and after noticing that she lacked many essential items, declared, "What's mine is yours. We can share everything."

This generosity, which is a lovely quality, had been hard for us to manage when trying to teach Suzy the boundaries she needed to implement in her life. Suzy saw Joan as a damsel in distress, and she wanted to alleviate some of her pain. Joan never learned to read and had a severe speech impairment, prompting Suzy to take her under her wing when she wanted to withdraw. She would take her by the hand to join her at social activities and in her most solicitous voice said, "This is my friend Joan. She is such a lovely girl."

Al and I became concerned that Suzy's growth was being stifled by her ceaseless desire to protect Joan, so we spoke to the dean at school, who did address our concerns and planned to widen the net. A social worker met with the two girls to explain how their interdependency was a hindrance to them both. It was suggested that they separate their time more and find their own interests. Suzy was invited to participate in activities that Joan was not cognitively able to manage. Joan was introduced to other students who were more like her and with whom she had a more equal relationship.

When Joan met another young lady who was not at all interested in including Suzy, Joan forgot about the loyalty she had been shown and moved on without Suzy. The idea of allegiance in this population is a difficult concept, and although we spoke about it frequently, it was hard for Suzy to understand, both then and now.

Suzy soon graduated to a new facility, which was comprised of four students living together with a house mother. She continued academic classes but also improved her life skills, such as laundry, cooking simple meals and basic cleaning (sweeping, washing dishes, vacuuming), and being more responsible for herself. Every time I visited, I was disturbed by what I perceived as a lack of cleanliness. Opening the drawers, I would see crumpled clothes and would begin to organize. Suzy would scold me: "Mom, stop, I folded it already." Because of her poor visual skills and impaired perception, her version of "folded" seemed twisted and askew. One day, Suzy must have seen the look on my face, and she shot out, "Mom, I see how hard this is for you. You can reorganize my drawers if it will make you feel better."

I began and then stopped, realizing the unfair statement I was making. I asked, "Suze, are you satisfied with the way your clothes are laid out?" When she answered that they were fine for her, I replied, "Excellent; this is your room and your clothes, and I am proud of all the effort you showed organizing your room."

The bigger lesson for me on that day and every day after was understanding that Suzy gives 110 percent to everything she does. Although I could continue to teach her, I had to modify my standards to live in her world. Her world was imperfect to me, but her independence and satisfaction with herself were more important.

When the school included Suzy in a ski trip to nearby Jiminy Peak, I had to be reassured that she could manage. Thinking about my daughter's limitations—balance, perceptual problems, impaired vision, inability to judge spatial relationships, amongst others—I could not imagine how she would stand on a pair of skis. But she was sold on the idea, and I made a parcel of ski gear to send up to her school. The weekend was an enormous success, with Suzy eventually moving slowly but steadily down the bunny slope after several hours of concentrated lessons. She was ecstatic.

I wasn't supposed to find out that Suzy and another girl had gotten lost on the mountain after they went to the dining lodge to buy a drink. The ski patrol had been deployed, but fortunately an older couple found them wandering around, realized their conundrum, and brought them down to the lodge. When I asked Suzy if she was afraid, she replied, "No, I knew someone would find us. I was more worried about you hearing that I was lost."

She achieved so many incredible accomplishments, and with each one, I allowed myself to filter back further into a normal life. Suzy participated in everything that was made available to her. She became a cheerleader and led her squadron to warm applause at the athletic competitions. She played soccer and occasionally scored a winning goal or defended her side with determination. Academically, she was progressing but was challenged with making changes or calculating the number of hours between one period and another. Contrarily, her acuity on a calculator and her ability to remember everyone's schedule was nothing short of savant level. One teacher compared her to a short-circuited electrical connection, where certain chips shone brighter to compensate for the dull bulb in another area. She never left her room without her calculator. On one occasion, as we were buying some supplies at the local supermarket in Amenia, the cash registers crashed. Suzy pulled out her machine and declared, "I'll save the day," enabling the clerks to tally up the customer's purchases and cash out the sales.

I received a call one day asking me to send up a complete set of riding garb, jodhpurs, boots, and a helmet. Suzy was going to start horseback riding. Al and I were terrified but were assured by the school that Suzy was capable.

Sometime after that, we were invited up to Maplebrook to watch a gymkhana in which Suzy was competing on her assigned horse, named Hippy. Seeing her in her smart riding outfit astride Hippy was one of the most heartwarming moments of her time at Maplebrook. When she won her event, cantering over low jumps, Al and I looked at one another with bewilderment, remembering her diagnosis at birth. In fact, I sent over a video to Dr. Gold, her pediatric neurologist, who after seeing it called me with these words: "When I watched Suzy cantering around the ring on a horse, Jane, I unprofessionally wept." He stopped there, with no need to say anything more. We both knew what it meant, and we silently shared our thoughts, our gratitude, and above all our amazement.

Suzy and Hippy had a wonderful career together. Her relationship with her horse is an endorsement of equine therapy for treating neurologically challenged individuals. Gail, the riding instructor, told me that Hippy behaved differently when he was around Suzy, whinnying to her when she would come down to the stables. She won the equestrian award at school, which was an extraordinary feat.

Suzy made many wonderful lasting relationships at Maplebrook, even becoming romantically involved with a boy named Eddie. I say "romantically," but not in the way of teenagers. This was a more immature attraction, similar to what twelve-year-olds would experience.

We were out to dinner one night with Eddie and his parents, who were glad that Suzy and Eddie were "dating." They felt she was a great influence, as she always encouraged him to participate in activities, be on time, eat nutritious food (he had gained fifteen pounds), call his parents, and so on. He made very little eye contact, and she did most of the talking, but when the topic of graduation came up, he immediately responded, "After graduation, Suzy and I will get married, and she will walk the dog, work, and take the garbage out!!"

I looked at Al and knew exactly what he was thinking. Suzy looked at us and without hesitation said, "Eddie, I think we should just be friends! I am not interested in marriage!" What a relief!

I had been concerned about them becoming sexually active, but Suzy assured me that she had no interest and stated with conviction, "Who needs that aggravation, Mom?" Eddie had many cognitive disabilities, and he was socially inappropriate, so we were thrilled when after a year, Suzy called us to say the relationship was over.

During her last two years at Maplebrook, Suzy moved to apartment living called "The Sky's the Limit." She lived somewhat independently with three other girls. In this step up, she was responsible for her time, schedule, hygiene, work, and social life. Support was available to ensure she was coping, but her daily life was hers to manage. Suzy had begun working at Astor Day Care and was ready at 6.00 a.m. every morning to ride the bus to school with the little ones. Her job included entertaining the children, observing their behavior, and making sure they were wearing their seat belts. The latter responsibility was extremely difficult for her, considering her poor fine motor skills, but she always managed and kept the children safe.

Al and I met with her coworkers. I beseeched them to be honest and give me a forthright answer about Suzy's work habits. We were emphatically told, "When Suzy isn't here, we are shorthanded." The more difficult the child, the more success she encountered, using her empathy, understanding, and lack of fear to confront a situation. Everyone strongly felt that her future was destined to be in childcare. She had become a valuable member of the day care team. She knew this was something she loved doing and would want to continue when she came home.

Then the unthinkable happened. Al came rushing home from work one day, urging me to pack an overnight bag, as we were on our way to Amenia. Obviously something was wrong, but he was being circumspect. Finally, he confessed that he had received a call from the hospital next to Maplebrook, telling him that Suzy was in the hospital, having been run over by a truck.

"Why didn't they call me too?" I said, panicked and needing to know more.

"Because Suzy made them promise they would not call you, knowing your reaction would be exactly what you are exhibiting now: sheer panic," he replied, slightly exasperated. "She has no broken bones but is badly shaken up, and we need to get up there as soon as we can."

We broke every speed limit on our way to the hospital. A nurse took us to the room Suzy was lying in. We didn't recognize our daughter. Every inch of her was black-and-blue. She had been very badly hurt but miraculously suffered no broken bones.

Even in a life-and-death situation, Suzy couldn't help defaulting to her compassion and forgiveness. In a woozy voice, she slurred, "Mom, don't be angry with the driver. He didn't see me. He felt terrible about what happened. He was the first person to call the ambulance and stayed with me until they came."

The accident took place at a notoriously bad blind spot on the road between her independent living and the school building. Everyone knew it would only be a matter of time before something like this happened. We petitioned for a traffic light to be put up at the pedestrian crossing, and this came to be known as the "Suzy light." It proved to be an enormous improvement in the safety of students. We were just grateful that Suzy had lived to tell the tale. I always felt that Suzy was put on this earth to improve the suffering of others but regretted deeply that her misfortune came at such a price.

Towards the end of her final year, Suzy was elected as the homecoming queen. Al and I were thrilled when we received an invitation to attend the event. Leaving Al to locate our table number, I went to find Suzy in her room, and together we decided between two sparkly dresses we had picked out. We chose the blue one, as it would twirl beautifully when she danced. Her hair and make-up had been professionally done, and she looked radiant.

The moment Suzy entered the hall, there was a thunderous applause. In typical Suzy fashion, she wanted to share her crown with everyone. When the dancing started, she refused to get off the dance floor for even one second. She was the belle of the ball, enjoying her freedom and expressing her joy through the movements of her body. With all the dancing and excitement, no one could have imagined that Suzy was struggling, but I felt something was wrong.

Because Suzy's birthday was July 18, less than three weeks after the cutoff date of June 30, we were incredibly fortunate to have the board of education continue to pay for her education at Maplebrook for an extra year. This meant she would graduate just shy of her twenty-second birthday, giving her a full five years as opposed to four.

Knowing how difficult it was going to be to find a replacement for Maplebrook, we began our research at the beginning of her last year. I had completely shifted my opinion about her living at home. We were all concerned about the transition from this wonderful environment, where she had made so many special friends as well as realizing her dream of living independently from her family. I realized that she flourished in an independent situation in her own world. I knew that wherever that was needed to be a little closer to us, but I had come around to understand what was best.

Graduation day was traumatic for Suzy. We sat in the audience, cheering her on, but I understood she didn't want to be in this position. She had had the opportunity to be her own person, and she was frightened to come home and be a little child again. I was frightened too, for I knew I would pick up where I left off—as an overprotective helicopter mom. I can't say that I wasn't looking forward to having Suzy geographically closer to us. How was I to balance my tremendous need to envelop her with my unconditional love and her own need for continued independence?

On the last day of Suzy's stay at Maplebrook, I was paralyzed with anxiety. Packing up her room and boxing the beautiful mementos, letters, accolades, and awards that Suzy had received over the years, I was overcome with sentimental sadness. She exemplified bravery and tenacity. Suzy couldn't bear to say goodbye to Hippy, to her friends and teachers, to the custodians, and all those in the village who had come to know and love her. I stood beside her, acknowledging this difficult transition and the uncertainty of the future. She was bravely offering positive encouragement to the other graduates, but I knew her heart was breaking.

Al and I had made certain decisions, but I wasn't convinced they were the right ones. Only time would tell. And there was something nagging at me. I was suspicious about Suzy's physical deterioration. That last year of school, she was very tired but kept pushing and pushing. I had often brought her home or gone up to her school for the weekend when she quietly let it be known that she didn't feel very well.

Sometimes we would be in town, and she would collapse with the effort of walking. I would find the closest motel and rent a room to let her rest. Instinctively I knew there was something very wrong, but I had no idea we were on the brink of the biggest battle of her life.

8

HERO

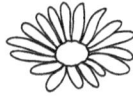

During the last year of Maplebrook, Al and I spoke to several of the other parents with graduating students about purchasing a house next to the school. The idea was to put a day care facility on the property and have the graduates operate the business while having a place to live.

Although the other families were wonderful, and the idea of creating a business of their own was enticing, my sixth sense told me that we needed to keep Suzy closer to home. Al and I had been told about Jespy House, which appealed to us for several different reasons. Jespy was started in 1979 with five adults who had aged out of the school system. Unfortunately, this population has not been accommodated once they are out of school, so with little outlet, the consumption of food becomes a hobby. The tendency to being overweight or obese is high. Without purpose, they languish, often in group homes, depressed, unhealthy, and unmotivated. The founders of Jespy wanted to change the future for their children with special needs. At its origins, it functioned as a daytime facility offering programs to provide stimulation and engagement. After this proved to be a much-needed asset to the community, overnights were introduced, and capitalizing on that success, large donations of money helped the purchase of the campus in which they are now. Over the years, with the help of private funding, including the Jewish Federation and the state of New Jersey, the vision has proven to be an invaluable service.

Al and I believed on many levels that this would be a good fit for Suzy. Located in the town of South Orange, New Jersey, it would keep her closer to us, but still allow her the independence she craved. With a cross-section of developmentally and intellectually disabled clients, Jespy provided a supportive alternative to promote self-direction, choice, and independent community living.

I found out that the director of special services during Suzy's Livingston public school days was now on the board of Jespy House. When I had originally started Parents and Professionals for Exceptional Children, he had not been a great fan of mine, as all my suggestions meant extra work for him.

The director insisted on having a member of his staff liaise with me and appointed Linda Halperin to the case. I think he secretly thought that Linda would be a watchdog and that we might butt heads, but to the contrary, our strong personalities melded beautifully. Linda had always been a strong advocate for people with special needs and now collaborated with me to become very vocal about the program. I was ardent about my goals and stressed the need for a socialization program, a vocational program, and a life skills program. With my relentless tenacity, I know I was a handful. Now I was afraid that when he saw my name as an applicant's mother at Jespy, he would refuse to even see us. But he was a terrific guy, and after his initial surprise, he was very receptive and friendly.

With my characteristic assertiveness, I went to see Jespy's administrative staff with a full list of requests and ideas for the long term. Although I knew they would accept Suzy without any problems, I still had to go through all the required steps, which once again meant producing all her records over the years. They approved her admission almost immediately, acknowledging her incredible social skills and aware that she would be a tremendous asset to their population.

As per the requirements, Suzy needed to spend the first year in the residential program. With a tremendous gradation in the caliber of the population, the staff needed to assess Suzy's capabilities. The range of support varied from one or two days per week to twenty-four hours a day. The more independent ones could live alone in one of the apartment buildings in South Orange, receiving reinforcement for the more complicated tasks. A few couples even married and lived together alone, yet still received client programming to monitor their basic requirements and help them to manage their homes.

I was very realistic about Suzy's abilities to live solo, convinced that it was unlikely she would ever be able to do so. Suzy loved the idea of Jespy, as did we, and she got ready for her new home. Nonetheless, our excitement was slightly marred by our consternation about Suzy's repeated exhaustion.

Suzy moved into Jespy residence the summer after her graduation from Maplebrook. The goal was to continue improving on the abundant skills she had learned at Maplebrook and adapt them to an even more independent situation. She was working at Temple Beth Shalom in the nursery school program, which she loved and where they valued her participation in classroom activities.

Suzy's appointed house mother at Jespy, a petite woman by the name of Renee, had become a dear friend and an advocate for her. She loved her fiercely, and I am grateful to her for her vigilance around Suzy during this worrying time. I would call her every day to enquire into Suzy's physical demeanor. I was sure that Suzy was ailing with something but could not pinpoint what was generating the weariness.

Jespy, on the other hand, was proving to be a fantastic fit. Suzy was sharing an apartment with three girls, and because she had already had the experience of being away from home, she was thriving. The staff assured me that although I may not have approved of the level of cleaning, she certainly had been taught the basics of keeping an orderly house. Her social skills were superior to those of the other girls, who were not fortunate enough to have had her exposure to new experiences. I got my daily updates from Renee, and they were glowing.

By now Suzy had made a lot of friends, and she was always rallying everyone to join her in a sport or new hobby. She was very popular with the staff of Jespy as well as the clients.

Hanukkah came, and Suzy celebrated with the kids at Beth Shalom. They made homemade potato latkes, they spun dreidels, and they lit candles each day at school. I put a menorah in Suzy's residence, and each night went over to join the girls to light the candles and eat some chocolate gelt (chocolate wrapped in gold foil).

Suzy loved all holidays, and this was one of her favorites. We had long ago stopped buying a little gift for each of the eight days of Hanukkah, but I know that Suzy wished we had continued that tradition. On the fifth night, Suzy stayed in her room, lying on her bed. I was surprised to find her there, knowing she would never miss out on the festivities for no reason. I went in to feel her forehead, but there was no sign of a fever. When she saw my concern, she pulled herself to her feet and came out into the living room to resume the candle lighting, but without the enthusiastic joy she normally exuded.

Renee pulled me aside and whispered, "Jane, I agree that there is something happening with Suzy. Perhaps schedule a visit to the doctor again. She is having trouble waking up in the morning, and she is sluggish walking out the door. In the afternoon when she comes back home, she lies down on her bed and stares at the ceiling. She cannot reach to take her shoes off and often falls onto her heavy coat without the strength to remove it. I'm worried about her."

I also was worried that something was seriously wrong with Suzy. I had noticed how exhausted she was, and while she never complained, I knew instinctively that she was ailing. Despite many doctors' visits and numerous blood tests there seemed to be no cause for her fatigue. Suzy would only mention in passing that she felt tired, which in her language meant that she felt terrible. Although she lived in the supervised housing, she would come home for dinners and family functions, and I would pop over to Jespy to say hello. Each time I saw her, I noticed a deterioration in her appearance and demeanor. She had lost her spark and seemed lethargic and low in spirits. I made a doctor's appointment for the first available date.

Christmas and New Year passed with the speed of lightning. Nothing eventful happened in our home or Suzy's, but she was gently excusing herself from coming over for family occasions, as she felt she was taking up too much space with not feeling well.

It was the beginning of 1999, and life in the Fischer household had evolved into a sweet rhythm of routine. Suzy had become invaluable in her job at Beth Shalom and was comfortably settled into Jespy House. Al and I had each assumed our varying parental roles, Beth was dating, and Ben was acting out his teenage angst. I was teaching, for a small salary but an excellent teachers' union medical insurance package.

I took Suzy to get her blood checked. The doctor told us she was slightly anemic, but nothing else was alarming. I wasn't convinced, but we followed the suggested protocol of taking iron supplements for six weeks. When we repeated the blood test, her hemoglobin was still 10.6, below the normal range of 12–16. The doctor blamed it on heavy menstrual periods and the possibility of Suzy not having taken the medication. But Suzy was always very conscientious about following instructions, and I knew there was no possibility that she had missed even one day.

I watched over Suzy during the next few weeks, returning to the doctor when I saw her getting worse over the following weeks. I didn't care that he felt I was being neurotic when he set up a visit with a hematologist to appease me.

The hematologist did an extensive blood workup, and when the news came, it was startling. Suzy meanwhile had started to complain about nausea. With some urgency and not without alarm, the hematologist told us that not only was her iron low, but she also had a creatinine range of 3.8. "What's creatinine?" I asked. My heart was in my stomach as I expected the next word to be *leukemia*. "Creatinine with an unusually high level is indicative of a malfunction in the kidneys," he continued. "Your pediatrician and I have already set up an appointment for a nephrologist to examine Suzy. The best-case scenario is that it might be something as simple as plumbing, but we want to rule out all other possibilities."

Although a nephrologist is simply a kidney specialist, *nephrologist* sounded like *executioner*. By this time, Suzy's fatigue took her to bed, and nausea kept her lying on the bathroom floor. Whatever was happening was getting more serious. The creatinine levels indicated the kidneys' inability to filter the blood and excrete toxins in the urine. The doctors were still somewhat optimistic in believing it might be a relatively benign issue, but the next step was a kidney biopsy.

We had had dark days with Suzy, but the day of the percutaneous kidney biopsy might have been one of the most gut-wrenching days of her life thus far. At 7 a.m. we arrived at the hospital, changed into hospital gowns, and covered our heads with paper caps. I was allowed to stay in the room, for although Suzy was chronologically twenty-four, she was still mentally ten and needed the comfort of her mom. There were four others present: the doctor, his resident, and two nurses. Suzy had not had anything orally for the eight hours proceeding and was very thirsty, but I could not give her anything to drink. She lay on her back while the doctor marked an area on the skin of her abdomen. The nurses began to disinfect the area and apply a numbing medication.

The room was icy. Suzy was shivering with cold, and I was shivering with the fear of the unknown and the complexity of the procedure. I hid my terror from Suzy with song. She was bravely waiting for the local anesthetic to begin to work.

The doctor approached her with a long 18-gauge needle. He identified the best point of entry into the skin and made a small incision. I held my breath and whispered in her ear, "There's a hero; look inside your heart. You don't have to be afraid." As the needle went further into an area too deep to have benefitted from the numbing agent, her body jerked with acute pain. I held her clammy hands, tears streaming down my face as the needle continued its journey in search of the damaged organ. The seconds turned to minutes, which, in extreme pain time, is hours. With every millimeter of tissue impaled during the probe, I sang louder: "There's a hero; look inside your heart. You don't have to be afraid."

Suzy whispered back at me: "Mom, you are always my hero. But I want this to end. It hurts so much." I was insane with helpless rage. I sang on and on, to both of us, searching for a mantra in the repetition of the words.

The doctor, aware of the horrendous pain he was inflicting, looked over at me with a gaze that offered compassion and apologies but also made me understand this was not yet over. He probed deeper, and the pain worsened. "I'm so sorry, Suzy, I'm so sorry. Another minute." The nurses rubbed Suzy's feet and legs, encouraging her to make it through.

Watching a child hurt is one of the most agonizing experiences a parent can have. When you can't stop it or fix it, it is the kind of heart-wrenching grief that you hope never to feel. The doctor was asking Suzy to hold her breath and, with a sharp clicking noise, he located the kidney and was able to collect a sampling of the tissue. He removed the needle, and the nurses covered the wound with a small bandage. We gave Suzy ice chips and told her the worst was over. I hugged her to me, letting her whimper into my neck. We were unable to articulate the trauma of the procedure, both of us aware that it would live with us for a long time.

During the recovery, Suzy continued to lie flat on her back, covered with weights that looked like sandbags. She had to keep from moving around for fear of hemorrhaging. They scrupulously monitored her vital signs—blood pressure, pulse, temperature, and breathing rate. Complete blood count and urine tests were ordered to ensure there was no internal bleeding. After an overnight stay, and once the vital signs were normalized, we were allowed to leave the hospital. The discomfort of the biopsy incision site was lessened with painkillers, but it would be some time until Suzy recovered from the ordeal.

The results took three days to arrive. We were hoping that it would validate the possibility of just some urethra blockage. At 9:00 a.m. on Monday morning, September 3, 1999, I was working as a learning consultant at Burnet Hill, a school for students with many different types of disabilities. I remember the phone ringing and the conversation that followed as if it were a minute ago: "Jane, the news is not good. Suzy has focal segmental glomerulosclerosis."

I asked the doctor to explain this foreign and portentous-sounding condition. "The glomeruli, of which there are thousands, serve as filters to help the body get rid of harmful substances; in this case, they are scarred and no longer able to function." Those shriveled little monsters had become deadly undercover assassins. "Suzy has only 12.5 percent of kidney function and is in the final stage of kidney failure."

What did he mean? I waited to hear the rest: "End-stage kidney disease is the last stage of chronic kidney failure, when the kidneys can no longer support a body's needs. This can result in death. Suzy will ultimately require dialysis and a transplant." I was also told that to get to the point at which Suzy was at, she would have been suffering for the last five years. The doctor urged us not to waste a minute.

My terror was audible. My girl—who so badly wanted to fit in, had pushed through barriers that any other person would have caved to. Since everything for Suzy has always been a struggle and a fight, she matured into a composed young woman, thinking that this unaccountable fatigue and nausea were just another evolution of the difficulties she had to endure. How I wish she hadn't been so stoic; we could have eliminated some of her suffering.

During each appointment at the doctor, they would ask her how she was feeling, and she would answer, "I'm OK, and how are you?" I would contradict her and say, "She is not OK." But Suzy did not give us accurate symptoms, so we could not define anything.

Our ignorance did enable Suzy to live a normal life longer than if we had been aware of her condition. Had we been alerted sooner, she would have been living at home with us on a low-protein diet, exercising, resting, and following guidelines that would not have changed the course of her disease but would have curtailed her quality of life. So in some ways, she enjoyed better subjective well-being during the years leading up to the critical point.

We took all the test results and the scans into New York for a second opinion, which was in accordance with the first. We drove down to my brother in Pennsylvania, and he had one of his pathologists read the reports, which correlated with the others. It had taken six months to ascertain the extent of what Suzy was up against. Now we were pushed up against a wall, navigating our way around this news. She was facing a life-and-death situation.

To prepare for the inevitable, Suzy was going to need a hemo-dialysis fistula to provide access to the dialysis. This procedure required surgery to join an artery to a nearby vein. The result was a larger subcutaneous blood vessel that could accommodate two needles. This kind of fistula is typically created in the non-dominant arm—the left, in Suzy's case—allowing her to use the right arm.

The doctor informed us that this was a forty-minute proce-dure. Al and I waited in the hallway. One hour went by, one and a half hours, two hours. Where was Suzy? Eventually, after four hours, the doctor came out, drained. "It was a very long and difficult operation, as Suzy has the veins of a small child."

When Suzy's creatinine clearance fell to 10–12 cc/minute, she was ready to start her dialysis treatments. Knowing this was not a cure for end-stage kidney failure, and with the understanding that clearing waste products and extra fluid from the body was a temporary although effective treatment option, we took her to the hospital outpatient center so she could be properly monitored.

Before, during, and after the treatment, all vitals were tracked very closely, and once a month, blood tests were assessed to ascertain the effectiveness of hemodialysis in removing waste from blood.

Not one treatment passed without an alarm sounding. Doctors and nurses would come running to check her issue, which was usually blood pressure or a blockage. After resolving the problem, they would be amazed when Suzy asked if she could go to work the next day. Despite her neurological challenges, Suzy was intuitive enough to understand how healing it was to remain employed.

In order to reduce the stress on the kidneys, we reduced her protein intake to four ounces a day. Her blood pressure was uncontrollable despite medication. Her anemia was getting worse, so they gave her infusions of Epogen, which works like the human protein called erythropoietin to help the body make more red blood cells. The doctors were very reluctant to have her receive any transfusions, as these would introduce antigens.

Suzy was the sunshine in the dialysis ward, the champion of optimism and hope for all the patients. When she arrived, you could hear her new friends calling her name with warm greetings: "Suzy, come over here and show me your new haircut." "Suzy, let's sit together today." Although she was the youngest patient, she forged wonderful, caring relationships. We always hoped that a special nurse, Sal, would be on duty as he was adept at finding her veins and he gave her much comfort.

One day, as Suzy was talking to her best friend, Sophie, she noticed her slump in her chair. "Sophie!" she screamed. "Sophie, why have you stopped answering me?" Sophie had been struggling of late, but now here she was, not responding.

There followed a catastrophic series of events with a code blue alert sounding loud and clear. Sophie passed away, only sixty-two years old, and Suzy was sure it would be her turn soon. "Why, mom? How could she die? Why didn't she get a kidney?" It was heartbreaking and traumatizing. After that, Suzy would shake when she walked into the dialysis ward.

The insurance company turned down our first request for home dialysis, but after reviewing letters from psychiatrists and other professionals, they compromised with the caveat that I would administer it. I could not agree to that. Even with the training I would receive, I would be ill-equipped to handle an emergency. We were eventually granted qualified nursing staff, and after rebuilding our basement with a specialized plumbing system, we hooked up the equipment at home. Timing was more flexible, we had two amazing nurses, and we waited for news on a donor.

Meanwhile, Suzy's kidneys deteriorated, and so did her quality of life—muscle spasms, nausea, high blood pressure—and yet Suzy found the will to endure.

From the minute we received the news about her condition, we had been on the hunt for a donor kidney. "Take my kidney," I fervently declared, unaware of the restrictions around organ donation. Suzy's blood type was O; mine was A; this could not be a match. Al volunteered his. Although he was blood type O, he was prone to kidney stones, which was not an option. We were all tested for human leukocyte antigens, which are proteins on the cells in the body. These tests ruled out Ben as a match, since his antigens were incompatible with hers. Finally, it was Beth's turn, but Suzy forbade us to even consider this option. Although the doctor had been talking over her head, she interrupted him, saying, "I will not take a kidney from my sister. She wants to have children soon, and I would never jeopardize her health to rule out that possibility." When Suzy put her foot down, no meant no. Beth insisted on pursuing testing, but after visiting several doctors, it was determined that she was not a suitable donor at that time.

We registered with UNOS (United Network for Organ Sharing). They have a national network of candidates waiting for and offering up organs. As in our case, willing donors are not always suitable matches, and it becomes necessary to search further afield.

UNOS optimizes the transplant system in the United States, ensuring that arrangements are handled ethically and safely.

To get Suzy's name on a waiting list for a transplant at a hospital, we had to go to each one individually, endure the test process over and over, and be put on a waiting list. New York hospitals had a seven-to-ten year wait, while at Jackson Memorial Hospital in Miami it was two to three years. At the time, the Florida motorcycle helmet laws were more relaxed, and because of the number of related accidents, donor organs were more available. As we moved about the East Coast, Suzy limped through the travels, by now in a seriously ill condition. Cell phones were not yet part of our lives, so each hospital gave me a beeper for immediate contact should they receive any news. How we longed to hear a beep!

With time now our mortal enemy, we were relentless in exploring every possible lead. Paying for organs in the United States is illegal, but as time went on, I began to consider doing anything to get my daughter a kidney. I learned that the black market for kidneys was robust, preyed on vulnerable groups, and violated every ethical consideration I embodied. Yet with desperate fear that we would not receive a kidney in time, I investigated the Dominican Republic as an option. I would have done anything to keep my baby alive. When we understood that the actual transplant would have to be done on-site in the DR, Al and I decided to hang on a little longer for the correct channels to produce results.

The journey to find a suitable kidney donor brought us many experiences, some beautiful and many harsh. One of the more extraordinary connections we made was with a wonderful woman, whom I'll call Anne. She was a good match and an eager participant. At the time of meeting her, Suzy wasn't yet below 12 percent functionality, and we couldn't do the transfer until it dropped.

Anne became part of our family, and we became part of hers. We established a remarkable friendship. She adored Suzy, and we found out that Anne was on a mission to "pay it forward." When she was a young girl, she gave birth to a baby out of wedlock, who was adopted by a family chosen by the nuns of her parish. Anne felt that by donating a kidney to Suzy, in some bizarre way she was redeeming herself. We in turn joined her on a quest to find her "baby," who, of course, was a grown woman now. We visited Anne and her family many times, spent holidays together, and cried together when her father passed away. We truly believed, in some divine way, that our bond was predetermined and a higher power had brought us together.

When the time came for the transplant, Anne had to undergo another round of testing. At this time, surprisingly, a lump was found in her breast, which turned out to be malignant. Imagine our shock and devastation. We gave Anne support throughout the testing and chemotherapy. Of course, she was eliminated as a kidney donor. Our pain was multifaceted, but of course both Anne and Suzy were our focus.

Anne passed away several years ago. It was a devastating loss, but for the time we knew her, she allowed us to believe in the kindness and generosity of the human spirit. I still speak to her mom and reminisce about the many heartfelt stories that we share.

We put an article about Suzy's plight in many local papers, including the community paper and *The Star-Ledger*, the paper that circulated throughout New Jersey. I received offers from prison inmates, pensioners, neighbors, family, and friends. No one was a match. As Suzy got sicker on dialysis, we became more and more desperate to find a donor.

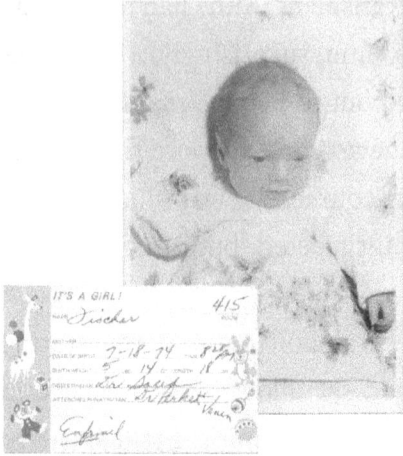

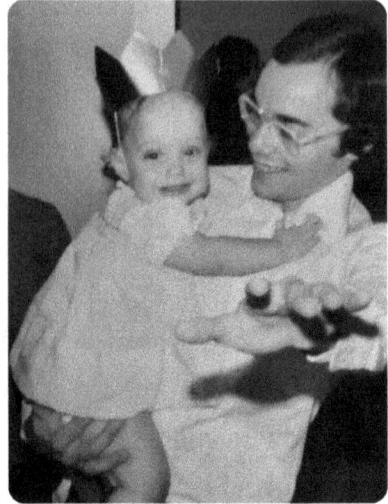

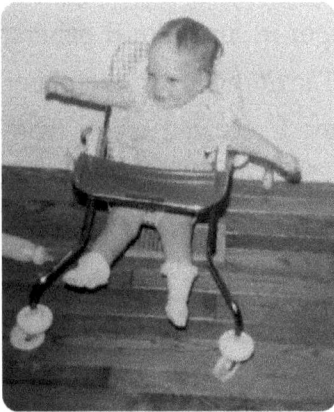

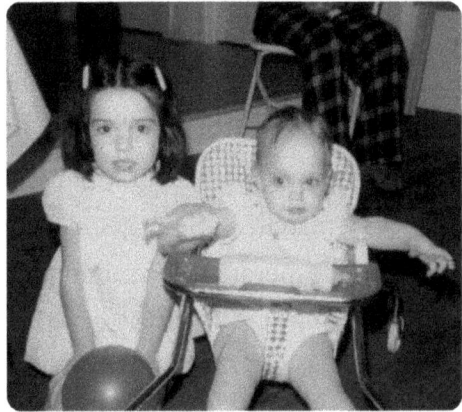

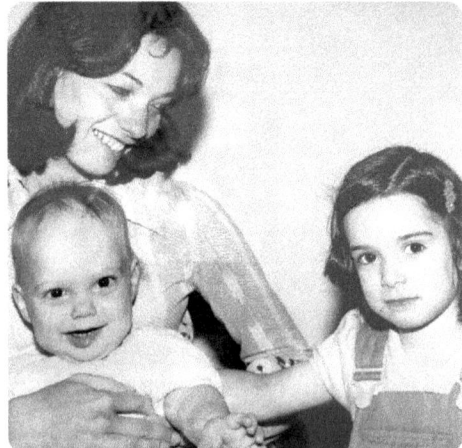

TOP LEFT: Suzy's birth
announcement.

TOP RIGHT: Suzy with Uncle Neal
at her first birthday party.

ABOVE LEFT: All smiles
in her walker.

ABOVE RIGHT: Beth and Suzy at her
first birthday party.

RIGHT: Jane with Suzy and Beth.

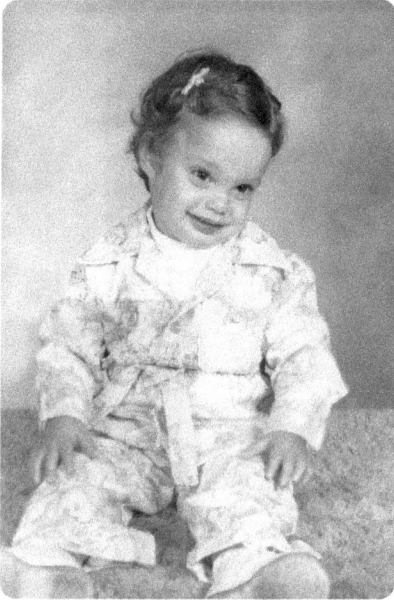

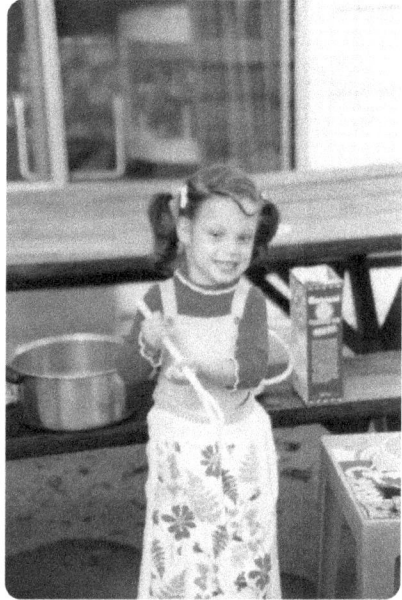

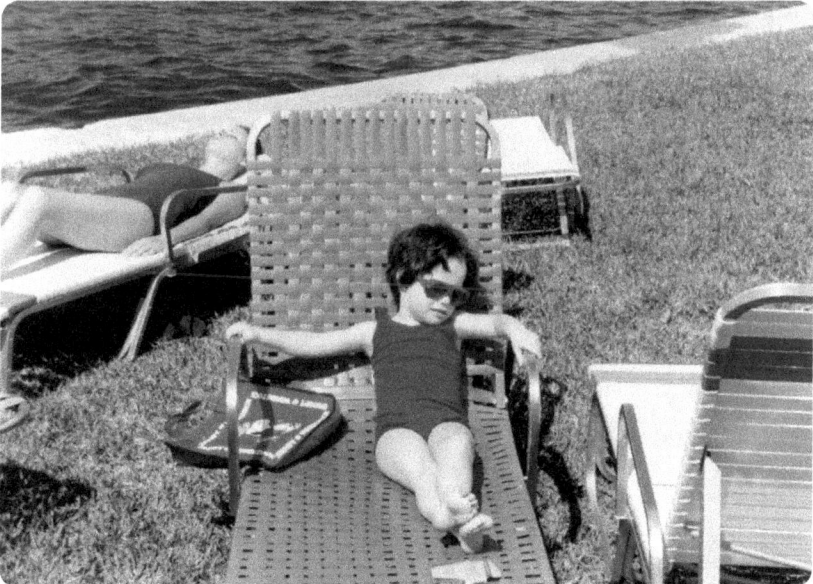

TOP LEFT: Suzy at thirteen months.

TOP RIGHT: In the kitchen with Suzy.

ABOVE: Four year old beach baby.

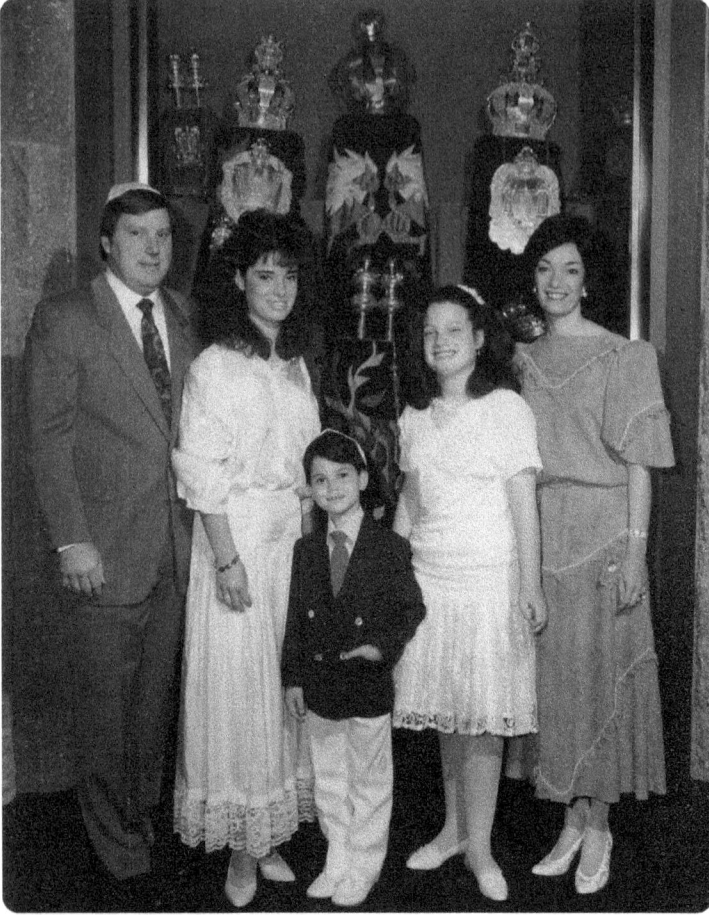

ABOVE: Suzy's Bat Mitzvah.

LEFT: Tournament of Champions

BELOW: Suzy and Jane at Maplebrook.

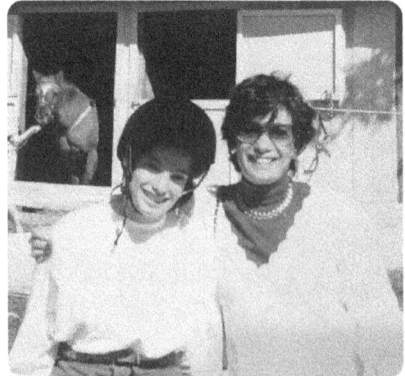

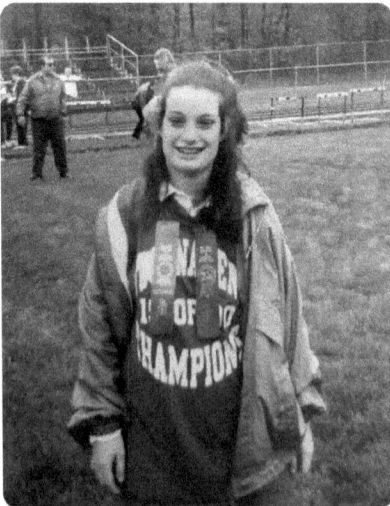

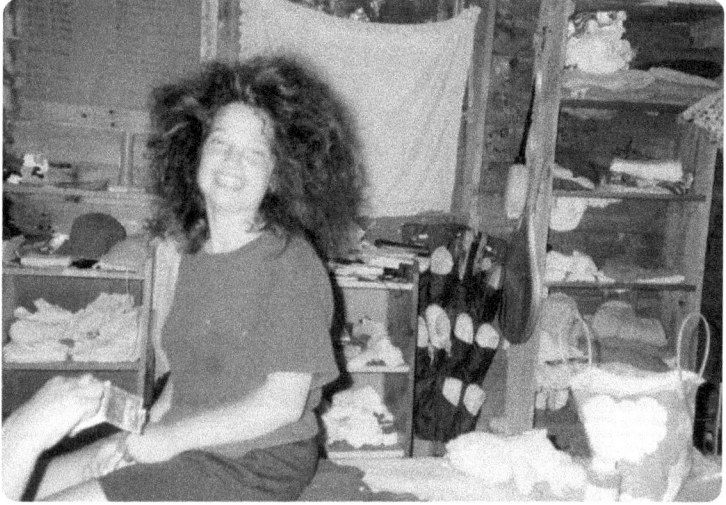

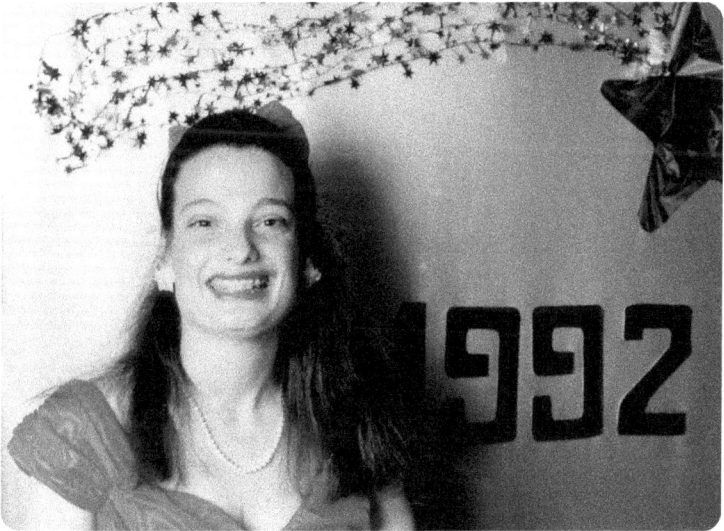

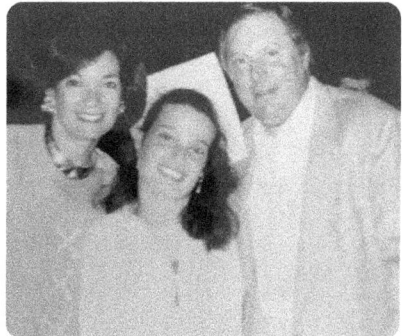

TOP: Camp Northwood.
ABOVE: Prom Queen.
RIGHT: Graduation from Maplebrook.

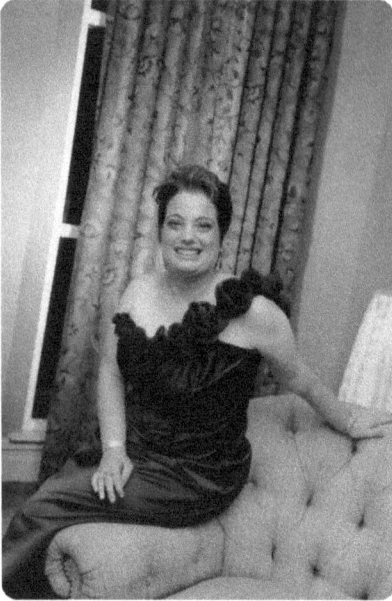

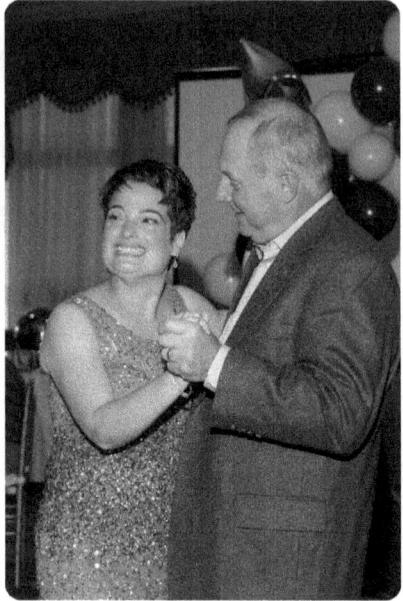

TOP LEFT: At Ben's wedding.

TOP RIGHT: Daddy's girl.

BELOW LEFT: Suzy at her condo.

BELOW RIGHT: All smiles even after her second kidney transplant.

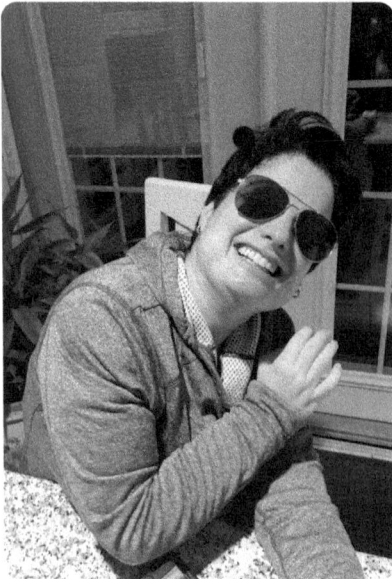

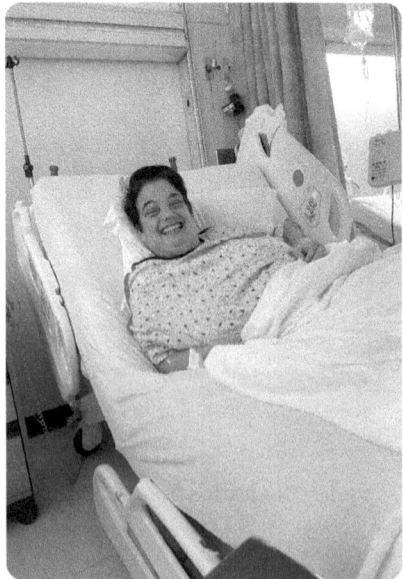

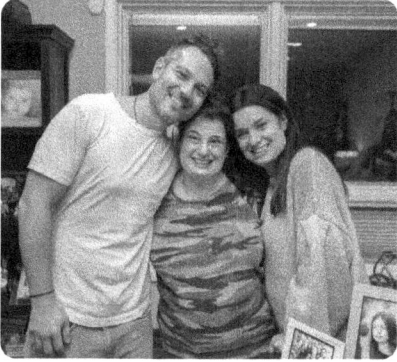

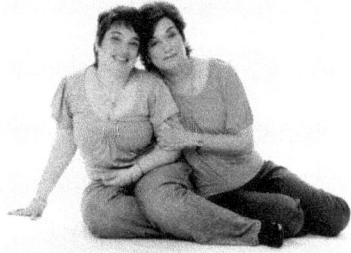

ABOVE LEFT: Ben, Suzy, and Beth.
ABOVE RIGHT: Suzy and Jane.
RIGHT: Suzy with Granny Bailey.

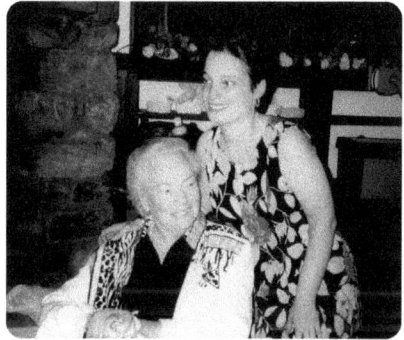

Andy Foster Photo

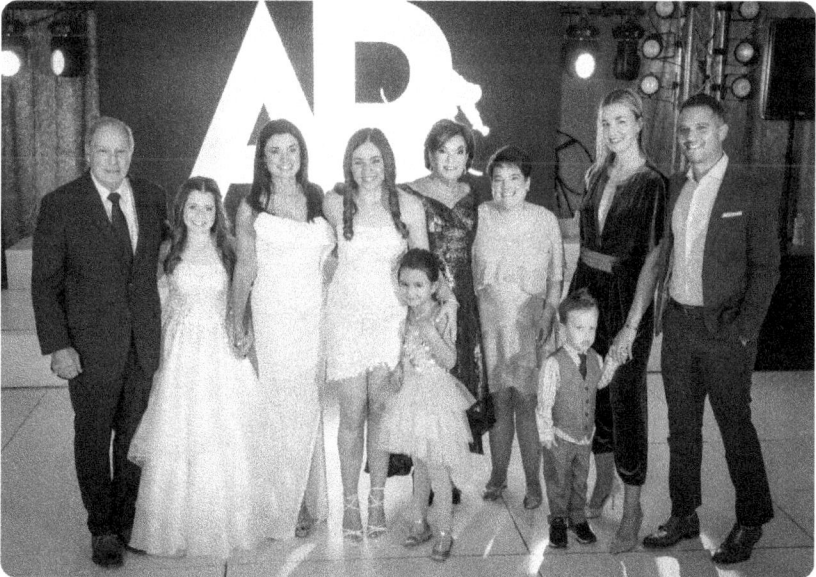

The whole family.
LEFT TO RIGHT: Al, Alyssa, Beth, Sydney, Bailey, Jane, Suzy, Cole, Britt, and Ben.

9

I WILL SURVIVE

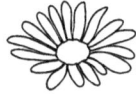

uzy continued to participate at Jespy as much as possible, but it was getting harder and harder. The director's twenty-two-year-old daughter, Jen Kutcher, became a companion to Suzy, developing a lovely friendship and introducing her to the world of art. With dialysis sapping Suzy's life, this was a wonderful distraction, although Jen, recovering from a difficult period in her own life, always felt that Suzy gave her more than she received. They nurtured one another with compassion and dignity through their difficult moments.

Feeling unwell most of the time, Suzy did have to come home a lot. We continued paying her tuition at Jespy, encouraging her to return when she could. Her spirits got a charge from being around her friends and having activities rather than thinking about her illness.

Hemodialysis required hospital stays up to four hours, three times a week, which interfered with Suzy's normal schedule. I considered switching to peritoneal dialysis. This method collects waste from the blood by washing the empty space in the peritoneal cavity by means of a catheter inserted into the abdomen. Although the doctor was willing to proceed with this measure, the side effects terrified me, and after much consideration, I felt it to be dangerous for Suzy. So we continued the long, boring days at the dialysis center, which meant Monday, Wednesday, and Friday were extricated from Suzy's calendar because of exhaustion and emotional upheaval.

Suzy was extremely ill during the procedures, and she had to miss a good six months of Jespy to remain isolated. She didn't want to stay at home with me hovering over her. She liked the attention, but she needed to breathe, away from my vigilance. She advocated going back to Jespy as soon as possible.

Finally, after two and a half years of being on a waiting list for a kidney, we were on the plane returning from a visit to Jackson Memorial Hospital in Miami, where Suzy was being evaluated for their transplant waitlist, when one of the beepers started going off. We thought it might have been due to the turbulence of the aircraft and had to wait to return home to call. At 9 p.m., as we were walking in the door, I heard the landline ringing. I ran to answer and heard, "Jane, I've been trying you for hours." It was Rachel, our case worker at Saint Barnabas. "We have a match for Suzy. It looks good." I started to ask some questions.

"Whose kidney, Rachel? Can I have the circumstances of the passing?" Rachel explained that the lady had died of a cerebral hemorrhage at sixty-three. She was the right blood type and had three of the six matching antigens optimal for the transplant. "A sixty-three-year-old kidney in Suzy, who is only twenty-four? How long is that going to be any good to her?" My excitement exploded, with valid concerns also tumbling out of my mouth.

Al took the receiver: "Let's have a moment to confer with Suzy's doctors and Jane's brother." We were given just ten minutes to decide, or they were going to reassign the kidney to someone else.

The donor had been declared brain-dead by four different doctors from four different disciplines, as is required by law. Since the organs would begin to break down without oxygenated blood, she was being held on life support.

My brother was the first to pick up the phone. "Jane, take the kidney. You don't know how long it will be before you receive another offer or whether you will even receive another offer. You have exhausted your options and your time. Call them back with a yes." Suzy's doctors agreed without hesitation, reminding me of the terrible problems Suzy was having with dialysis.

We had no time left to dither. Her veins had all but collapsed, the fistula was raw, and her heart badly affected. She never came off the machines without alarm bells ringing.

We were at the hospital by 10:30 that same night. By 4 a.m., the preop testing was completed, and they wheeled Suzy down to dialysis. We had been traveling for two days, and she was overdue. Since she was so sick, I was afraid they would refuse to operate.

Suzy had been taking strong doses of prednisone, cyclosporine and Prograf, the most recognizable of the immune suppressant drugs. By destroying her immune system, they increased her chances for a successful transplant but could also enable a small cold to turn into pneumonia.

I wrapped my sweater around my arm to conceal my nervous shaking. Watching my daughter going into a life threatening surgery was so emotionally confusing. I had to believe that she would survive and thrive, but I also understood the risks. Despite sounding upbeat as I kissed Suzy goodbye, she could read my fear. Grabbing my hand, Suzy whispered in my ear, "Mom, I love you so much. Be strong."

Both Suzy and her donor's kidney were wheeled into the operating room. The donor had been kept alive until such time as the transfer could take place, as the kidney would only remain healthy for thirty-six hours on life support. Any longer, and the tissues would deteriorate, rendering the organ useless. We were under the time limit, but only just. Cadaveric donor identities are kept a secret, so I never knew the woman who was Suzy's savior.

The doctors began the five-hour operation. We sat outside the operating room, unable to read or even converse. I remember how complicated my emotions felt around my daughter receiving a kidney from a deceased person.

Al didn't always have the most uplifting skill set, but I was grateful for his company in the cold corridor and appreciated him deeply when he wrapped me in his cardigan and brought me hot coffee. He was a rock, albeit a stubborn one, with jagged edges.

I rolled back my life and examined the trajectory that had brought us to this surreal moment. We had had some bad luck, but we were first and foremost a family with the right principles. My parents had given me the tools to be warm-hearted and gentle, but it would be my three wonderfully different children that unwittingly gave me strength and force. They would forever be the most significant influences in my life.

Glancing down at my watch, I felt lightheaded with hope. It had only been an hour, and I was already racked with anxiety about the outcome. I needed to get outside, away from the clinical corridor with its antiseptic odor. I took the elevator down to the first floor and took some deep breaths in the fresh air. I looked up in the sky, perhaps expecting to see a message written on a cloud, or even the specter of God.

I checked in with myself in the cold December air. A woman with a small child hooked up to breathing apparatus in a wheelchair stopped to ask me the direction to the pediatric cancer ward. Hospitals are grim reminders that many parents are dealing with very sick children. I wanted to say something appropriate but just pointed to a building in the next quadrant.

The unfairness of life's lottery had knocked me down. I thought of the old adage, "Throw everyone's problems in the air, and you prefer to catch your own." Although I hated to watch my daughter suffer, how grateful I was to have her in our lives!

I felt the chill now edging into my extremities and went back upstairs. My watch showed three hours since we said goodbye to Suzy. I visualized the surgery as it had been described to me. I saw the knife start under her breast slicing open her torso all the way to her pubis. Choosing to leave the original kidneys in place shaves hours off the surgery, as getting to them would require more cutting. The donor organ, about the size of a fist, was to be placed into the right side of her torso area, and the blood vessels of the new kidney attached to blood vessels in the lower abdomen above the legs. The final stage would be the attachment of the new kidney's ureter to the bladder.

Al was calling my name. I had slumped in the chair, and Ben and Beth had arrived without my realizing it. They ran over to sit next to us, bringing a new energy to my musings. They helped pass the time, and when I looked at my watch next, Suzy had been in the operating room for five hours and fifteen minutes. I stood up, willing someone to come out and give us some news.

I didn't have to wait long. The surgeon pushed open a door at the end of the corridor and with a tired smile said, "It's finished. It was a successful transfer. Suzy is doing well. Her blood pressure is a little high, but she is making urine already. We will have constant nursing care watching her condition." My little fighter had survived another battle.

But I didn't anticipate the severity of the aftermath. Suzy had been on the transplant floor about five days when she became unresponsive to her environment. Although her eyes were open, she stared into nothing, appearing to be in a coma. Emergency teams filed in around her bed, each one adjusting tubes and wires, adding sensors, testing her vital signs, and shouting instructions to one another. Al and I watched the action with our backs to the window ledge, which was the only thing that stopped me from sliding down the wall in panic. For twenty-four hours, we held our breath, wondering if we were losing her, until, as suddenly as it had happened, it stopped, and her condition stabilized. Not one professional could figure out what had happened. It could have been that she was dialyzed too quickly in the rush to get to surgery and she lost too much fluid from the brain. It could have been due to the monster dose of eighty milligrams of prednisone. It could have been from the anesthesia. We stayed in the hospital another week with constant surveillance around Suzy and, often, a nurse kindly making sure that I was composed.

When we were released from the hospital, we came home to fanfare and celebrations from afar. No one could get close to Suzy for fear that she would catch something. The body doesn't understand that the transplanted organ is saving a life, so it will attack, considering it a genetically foreign agent. We had to be extremely careful that she was not exposed to any germs. Beth and Ben could only stand at her bedroom door to talk to her. Al too. They were all continuing with their lives and exposed to the outside world, so it was my job to stay home and stay healthy to be able to care for Suzy.

On the next round of tests, we were told that her creatinine levels were rising again. She was having acute rejection of the new kidney despite the immunosuppressive therapy. We went back to the hospital, where she received intravenous doses of ganciclovir, an alternative to the previous cocktail. The doctors were hoping that it would be more effective in halting the rejection. At the same time, it would shut down her immune system completely, leaving her dangerously vulnerable to any infection.

The doctors suggested that I plan to stay alone in the room with her, eliminating all contact with the outside world. Any innocuous germ or virus could have killed her. As the rejection started to slow down, Suzy was reintroduced to the "triple threat" therapy of prednisone, cyclosporine, and Prograf. The recovery took over two months, during which time we remained isolated at home.

Suzy never felt well. Her creatinine level never dropped below 2.8, which was high for her. She was off dialysis, but the new kidney was never a good fit. She pushed through years of constant fatigue, low stamina, and multiple visits to the hospital when she was felled by an infection.

Although the transplant was a miracle of sorts, it was also fraught with many complications. As a result of the many meds, Suzy became a steroid-induced diabetic, developed chronic high blood pressure, high cholesterol, muscle spasms in her hands and feet, and cataracts. In addition, she got gout, urinary infections, and, most debilitatingly, an episodic severe cough that was triggered by any germ, any environmental debris, or often unknown origins. She suffered for weeks at a time with a relentless, continuous cough that plagued her day and night.

We went all over seeking medical opinions—Columbia, Cornell Weill, Mount Sinai, University of Pennsylvania hospitals, and we even flew to the Mayo Clinic in Jacksonville, Florida. Suzy was hospitalized for countless tests that yielded nothing, although the doctors hypothesized that the immunosuppression drugs had caused this atypical asthma, however nothing was ever conclusive. She was treated with nebulizers, additional steroids (which caused her sugar to go through the roof), humidifiers, antibiotics, and lots of codeine. Nevertheless, these coughing episodes had a mind of their own and lasted until they finally burned out on their own accord.

Once more we lived the truth of what we were told at our first transplant meeting: transplants are a treatment, not a cure.

Soon after Suzy had received her first kidney, she was asked to be a spokesperson for a program that was being set up in Essex County, New Jersey. Jim Treffinger was the Essex County executive who initiated Workplace Partnership for Life, an organ and tissue donation awareness initiative. Jim had heard about Suzy from an employee who had attended a talk I had given on the importance of organ donation. This young woman was so moved by Suzy's plight that she felt it was an important story to share. As the poster child for this initiative, Suzy was invited to give a talk about what it was like to wait in failing health to receive a donated organ. Her description was instrumental in educating the general public on the importance of organ donation.

During one of Suzy's many hospital stays, it was decided that she needed a colonoscopy. Later that night, Suzy became very agitated. She told me the IV pole was Ernie and Bert from *Sesame Street* and urged me to leave the room before the bad guys could catch me. These severe hallucinations continued through the night. I had no experience with psychotic episodes, refusing to believe that she needed to be given an injection of haloperidol, a medication that works in the brain to treat schizophrenia. Haloperidol rebalances dopamine to improve thinking, mood, and behavior.

I became unreasonably hysterical, and at 5:00 a.m., Al was summoned to come and take me away or reason with me to calm down. Suzy continued screaming that the police were coming to take her away because she was such a terrible person, and she would not let me near her because she did not want me to get hurt.

Everyone was yelling, tugging, and shrieking. The nurses from other stations asked us to quiet the noise, but we couldn't. Suzy was a furious demon, channeling Regan MacNeil in *The Exorcist*. Her rantings became louder and more intense as the danger she was seeing came closer.

I eventually realized that I could not control this situation and that Suzy was becoming dangerous to herself and perhaps even to me. I allowed them to sedate her. The haloperidol immediately calmed her and let her sleep. I wish they could have sedated me. Instead, I watched over my fragile daughter with the steady gaze of a hawk on a nest, talons ready to unleash on anything I decided was an enemy.

In 2003, Jespy awarded Suzy with the Profile in Courage award as a "a commendable pillar of the community who demonstrates courage under pressure." The Profile in Courage award perpetuates John F. Kennedy's legacy as a civic pillar for courage under pressure as well as everyday courage. Suzy was chosen to receive the award for her unfailing support of other people trying to conquer their adversaries while enduring countless obstacles and hardships herself. Suzy, by her example, personified the distinct message of this award.

I helped Suzy prepare her acceptance speech and was astonished when she rose from her seat, calmly and with poise, to walk onto the dais and address herself to a room full of well-wishers. I swelled with pride, reflecting on our journey together and marveling at what Suzy had achieved.

In 2004, we detected a nodule in Suzy's neck. A biopsy determined that she had thyroid cancer. Naturally, there was disagreement on how we should proceed, but after extensive exploration, the pathologists at the University of Pennsylvania felt strongly that the thyroid must be removed. The doctor assured Suzy that she would have a very small scar. Instead of panicking, she said, "Don't worry. I can always wear a pretty necklace to cover my neck."

We went through this new health crisis like young soldiers in basic training: follow the rules, stand tall and straight, obey the sergeants, and build trust in your team. Ben was graduating from college in June of that year, and we were of course all scheduled to attend. Suzy had a high threshold of pain, but this recent biopsy had been grueling. I knew how much pain she was feeling, but her priority was to make this day very special for her brother. When I checked in on her comfort, she would answer in an irritable voice, "Don't you dare say anything. Stop focusing on me. Ben deserves to be celebrated." Suzy, with IQ test results that got her turned down more often than I cared to think, had the heart of an elephant. She wanted no fuss. Her selflessness became legendary and often challenged me to consider my own. "Thank you, darling, you are correct. This is Ben's moment. I promise not to bring up your health."

Suzy attended the weekend celebrations as if she had had a clean medical slate her entire life instead of being a girl who flirted with death.

Her surgery followed in August, and at that time, we all rallied to share the responsibilities of the radiation that followed.

Naturally, a few new doctors and nurses who were administering the treatment were welcomed into the fold, having found Suzy to have a magnetic energy that trapped their hearts.

When Suzy was undergoing the therapeutics around her cancer, I was working full time and finding it challenging to monitor her saltless diet, attend to my ailing mother, and be a wife to Al and a mother to Ben and Beth. I was exhausted, but the medical insurance plan that I was given as a teacher was irreplaceable and helped us enormously with our bills around Suzy's relentless health issues.

I was working as a substitute teacher, having decided to go back to school in 1989 to get a master's degree in special education as well as a certification as a learning consultant. It was important for me to earn this qualification, and I was lucky to work with very understanding colleagues, who would cover for me when a crisis occurred. Coincidentally, the same year I graduated with my degree, Beth graduated college, and Suzy graduated from ECLC. We all wore our caps and gowns for a photo that was published in the local paper.

For Suzy, the worst part about being sick and needing to be isolated was her removal from daily routine and interactions with people. As soon as we could safely expose her to the general public, she returned to her jobs. One of her favorite positions was at my sister-in-law Judy's dental practice, where she had been working since she was seventeen years old.

One day, she was sitting at the front desk and recognized a patient. "Sam, I just mailed you a bill. You owe Dr. Post some money." Sam turned around to look at her in embarrassment as she indiscreetly announced this news in a crowded waiting room. Suzy was so earnest in her communication that it was hard to criticize her when these incidents occurred, so I was always treading a line between being tough and making allowances. When I chastised her, her face would crumple, and she would feel the weight of having displeased me.

Suzy wanted the world to be a better place and saw herself as a mentor and a teacher. In these roles and without the filters that we exercise to remain appropriate, she tended to be overreaching and invasive. Our family was forgiving, although there were certainly explosive moments when one of the kids would say in frustration, "Suzy, this is none of your business. Stay out of it." Suzy would be sad but bounced back quickly, offering a humorous comment on the situation, and reminding us all that she is the survivor, not the victim. She never stopped trying to be the best version of herself and was capable of being introspective and willingly accepting constructive criticism.

I would watch these interactions with conflict and sadness. Suzy was always more comfortable in her own world of people with special needs, where she moved more calmly and with more confidence. Within these environments, she was indeed the leader and facilitator she wished to be.

She never forgot the people who helped to make her life more palatable. One Thanksgiving, she worked with her basic skills teacher for weeks to create handmade, personalized greeting cards to express gratitude to the special people in her life. The list was endless! The project was difficult for Suzy, but she worked for weeks, patiently approaching the challenge with stubborn tenacity.

10

BE OUR GUEST

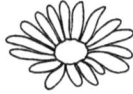

When Suzy showed signs of being a little better, I knew we needed to let her return to her housing at Jespy. Renee, our beloved friend, was still working there, so I felt confident that she was watching over her and would alert me to any emergency health situation that might arise.

Although Suzy should have been eligible to move onto a different category of housing at Jespy, the staff had been unable to evaluate her capabilities since she had missed so much time because of her illness. It became apparent that she would have to remain in the residential housing program until further notice.

I was immersed in the survival of Suzy and had little time for anything else. Ben, Beth, and Al never complained about my being out of touch with them, but I know I was very distracted, exhausted, and scared. It must have been terrifying for them to watch Suzy fighting for her life, and disappointing not to have extra hugs from me. I was always feeling guilty, as if I could never do enough for anyone. Lying in bed at night, my mind raced with thoughts of how I could be more available for all of those I cared for so dearly. I berated myself, wishing I had the arms of an octopus, able to reach out and touch all my loves.

Renee was calling me several times a day, not as an alarmist but as a genuinely caring friend and caregiver. Suzy's sugar was often too high, as was her blood pressure. I was running back and forth to Jespy, which fortunately was only twenty minutes away. I shuddered, thinking that she might have been in Amenia, three hours away. I thanked my intuitive self every day for making the right decision to have her closer to us.

Jespy was amazing. The administrators, Lynn Kutcher, Lisa Jasinski, and Lois Rose, assisted Suzy in every way, making her life as comfortable as possible. She inspired many of the clients and staff members with her pure goodness.

One day, Suzy was walking around and saw her computer teacher, Tim Raymond, apparently feeling a little down. As she greeted him with her usual warmth and friendliness, Tim noticed this huge swelling in her upper arm above her elbow, which was red, irritated, and looked extremely uncomfortable. Suzy asked him why he seemed so down. He was taken aback because here she was, with this awful fistula, but concerned about him. He called me, choking up, as he described how she showed him such loving concern while immersed in her own discomfort. It was the best antidepressant he had ever taken.

I, however, was contemplating a new plan. I could see that Suzy was never going to be living on her own. Not only did she have the cognitive issues, but now she had chronic health issues. It would never be safe to leave her unsupervised. I considered buying a home close to Jespy, which Al and I would finance and Suzy would live in, while renting out rooms to three other girls.

Al thought I had lost my mind, and in retrospect perhaps I had. It wasn't the best idea financially, but for reasons that I couldn't imagine or calculate at the time, I convinced my husband. "Al, it is so important for Suzy to think that she will have her very own place and that we believe in her recovery and long life span. I'm willing her to believe she can beat the odds. Perhaps a home of her own will psychologically give her the drive to find new strength. I understand this is not a sound financial decision or a clever business proposition, but it's an emotionally significant one."

I don't know where I found this conviction to argue with Al. I know I couldn't have argued like this for myself, but when it came to Suzy, I was possessed with the strength of titans and the bravery of a firefighter running into a burning building. Al, bless his heart, argued bitterly with me, but when I found the perfect four-bedroom home, he came around to believe I was correct, and we purchased it.

Al was exceptional when it came to allowing me to make so many of the decisions around Suzy's well-being even when he thought I was foolish. He gave me enormous rein in my role as captain, his unwavering support giving me a sense of solidarity.

Jespy, with a long waiting list of clients, needed Suzy's spot. Bringing her to live at home felt like surrendering to her illness, not to mention tapping into her worst nightmare. Even so, this was a wonderful solution, and I was grateful that we were able to facilitate it.

Before I could finalize the deal on the house, I needed a tacit agreement from Jespy that they would run the home as an extension of their program. They agreed to my terms, although everyone thought I was unrealistic, considering how ill Suzy was.

I trusted Suzy to make sound choices when living there, knowing of course there was always going to be twenty-four-hour help on call. For the first time, Suzy would not need to share a bedroom, and neither would her roommates. Suzy had the master bedroom with her own bathroom—a luxury she had not had before.

The house, an old Victorian built in the 1860s with original crown molding all around the ceiling, was charming. With four bedrooms, one for each girl, plus an additional bedroom off the kitchen, where the house mother could live, it felt like a little sorority house. I thought we could decorate it in pink and white. I wanted to keep the feeling of the era, so we started researching furniture that would work with the period. Suzy rallied from a hospital stay, and the two of us went shopping together. She loved the process of choosing couches, rugs, beds, kitchen accessories, and lamps. She had her definite preferences but allowed me to overrule her on some of the more outlandish ones.

The extreme dread from days of being hospitalized evolved into long shopping trips at the mall. We often brought home samples of fabrics and set them out on the kitchen table so we could test out combinations and designs. We looked at paint colors for the interior walls and then for the exterior. I wanted a three-seater couch and two armchairs for the living room, but Suzy wanted a sectional. I was able to convince her that they didn't have sectionals in the 1800s, so it wouldn't look authentic. I soothed her over by giving her carte blanche on the throw pillows and that is how we landed up with one mustard, one purple, and one red pillow. We kitted out the kitchen with pots and pans, crockery and cutlery, glassware, and the essentials like a toaster, a kettle, a vacuum, and a garbage pail.

Al installed a large kitchen clock so the girls would know what the time was. We sourced plants for the little garden and special lights that would come on automatically when you walked up the entranceway. We decided on curtains rather than blinds and we opted for comforters rather than duvets. Since there were no structural changes to be made, we were able to finish the interior to the point of being able to live there within a month. I figured that accessories could come slowly and could be an outing for the girls as they could go to a weekend flea market and rummage through the bargains.

Suzy was as proud as a peacock. Aside from decorating, she was looking forward to inviting the other ladies to join her in her home. We had been working on the list of roommates that Jespy had suggested and made our offers to the girls. We deliberately kept the rent affordable so that some of the less privileged girls could take advantage of the situation. We felt it was important to share our good fortune with others in the special-needs community, knowing how blessed we were.

The first group included Diane, who was a good friend of Suzy's from the residence. Having been born with cerebral palsy, she needed constant help with mobility. She relied on Suzy's unfailing optimism to help her through dark times. Cognitively, she was stronger than the other girls but was less confident, so her morale needed bolstering. She and Suzy remained friends even after the house was sold.

There was Kimberley, who had a higher academic level than Suzy but was not as social or outgoing. Suzy had a positive influence on Kimberley by including her in all the activities outside of the house. Kimberley was prone to remaining in her room, but when Suzy announced she had signed the two of them up for an event, Kimberley would enthusiastically tag along.

The last one, JoAnne, was a rabbi's daughter. She was a great candidate, but she didn't have the funds to pay the rent. We felt strongly about being able to offer her a place. While Al and I were reaching out to the community for donations, Suzy read my mind and announced, "Let's have a fundraiser." How did she even understand this concept? "I've been to other fundraisers, and it makes me happy knowing I am doing something for someone else." My daughter was all heart—love and giving. She only knew one way to behave in the world, and that was with pure, unbelievable generosity of spirit.

Having reached out to several sources, we were able to provide housing for JoAnne. We watched her blossom from a shy young girl to an extroverted woman with the security and support of her friends in the house. She had come from a large family of nine children, where it was often difficult for everyone to get their quota of attention. Here in the house, the girls nurtured her and gave her the wings to flourish, so that several years later, when she moved to a group home, she was talking, laughing, and interacting in a way she never had experienced.

Suzy had a home of her own and with that the pride of home ownership. She continued to suffer with her health, but blossomed into a beautiful innkeeper, ensuring the girls felt comfortable and completely at home. I knew she would be spending time in the hospital and at our house with her ailments, but she would also understand that we believed she would be well again and would not have to live in an institutionalized environment.

After the first few months in the house, Renee suggested a housewarming party for the girls and their parents. When we arrived, we noticed a huge card attached to the front door. It was a beautiful thank-you note, written by the girls and their parents, expressing their sincere gratitude for this opportunity. It was a dream come true for them and for us, as we all worried about the same issues. We cried and exchanged hugs, understanding the lonely nights of worry that we shared. For Al and me, being able to share our good fortune was the greatest gift we ever enjoyed.

After desserts and refreshments, Suzy and the girls asked us to find a seat and surprised us with a rendition of "Friends." They were all off-key, many words were incorrect, and they swayed in different directions, but it was the most moving rendition that I have ever heard. Al hugged me tightly, whispering, "All the hours of sweat and toil were worth it. We have been blessed to be able to bring joy to this cadre of young women. This is the meaning I ascribe to my life—sharing, community, generosity, and love." I looked over at him, puzzled to hear him say these words, proud that he was able to.

One night, I wanted to bring Suzy some snow gear, because a calamitous storm was predicted. When we rang the bell, Diane answered the door, and the scene before us warmed our hearts. The girls were eating dinner in the dining room under Renee's supervision. It was like a scene from *Little House on the Prairie*. Already in their pajamas, these four girls, each afflicted with various disabilities, were conversing and enjoying a family-style get-together like any evening we would have wanted for our children. While their conversation was not as sophisticated as that of our neurotypical children, the concern they felt for one another was evident in their faces and voices. Suzy was in full swing as the hostess and invited us to stay and have a cup of tea. We reluctantly refused, saying we did not want to interrupt, but all the girls insisted we stay to try their world-class Jell-O.

As the weather became worse, we asked Suzy if she might want to come home because of the predicted snowstorm.

"Absolutely not," she declared. She was going to stay and hang out with her friends. They had planned the games, chosen the movies, and were ready for anything. Renee assured us she would be there through the night. As it happened, the storm brought several feet of snow and a blackout around 10 p.m., as they were getting ready for bed. I had equipped the house with a couple of flashlights for just such an emergency, and Suzy made sure everyone got to their rooms before she made her way to her own.

The next morning, we banded together to plow out the entranceway, which was frozen and icy and could have proven hazardous if the girls had tried to walk over it. They all took the event in their strides, enjoying the excitement of the unexpected. A day later, if you had driven past the house, you would have seen a life-size snowman, which the girls had created together with Renee and me.

The house was starting to require intense maintenance. Diane had accidentally pulled the railing off the staircase as she struggled to get upstairs. Kimberley had become seriously depressed and needed more intense care. She was replaced by Phyllis, who had severe cognitive delay and whose decision-making was questionable. She stayed for several years until her parents felt she needed more supervision. JoAnne was able to stay in the house for seven years, but when the scholarship money ran out, her parents had an opportunity to place her in another facility that accepted her without cost.

One rather harrowing event occurred when the aide who was supposed to work till midnight decided to leave an hour early. This meant that the lady who was coming on duty for the graveyard shift had to ring the bell to be let in by one of the girls. Suzy heard the bell ring and went to the front door to open it. She has always been blissfully unaware that danger lurks, so it didn't occur to her that the person on the other side of the door might not have had good intentions.

One goal in Suzy's development was to foster independence, but consequently she thought she could do more than she could. On one occasion, the toilet became clogged. Suzy had watched me plunging toilets and was convinced she would be able to do this task on her own. So she plunged and she plunged and she plunged until the toilet broke and the bathroom, which was on the second floor, leaked all the way down to the basement. When the plumber came, he told us this could have been avoided had the toilet not been tampered with so aggressively.

One of the biggest issues was staffing the house. Even though Jespy was supposed to be monitoring this, I felt the full responsibility of making sure it went smoothly. It never did. One of the house moms stole from the girls. Another one left the girls alone in the house for several hours. Although we owned the house, we never wanted to be employers, and the pressure and worry were overwhelming. Matters such as a washing machine breaking down or toilets clogging became my concern as a landlord, and I felt I spent hours a week worrying about maintenance issues.

In 2019, after we had owned the house for thirteen years, we were asked by Jespy to put in a $100,000 elevator to accommodate Diane. We knew then that we had to sell and make alternate arrangements for Suzy. It had been a beautiful experience, but its time was over.

Although Suzy's health remained at best unstable, she wanted to live in her house as much as possible. While she was there, she had many friends and even developed a relationship with a chap named Richard. He was not a particularly suitable beau, as he relied on Suzy to provide the mothering. Their relationship became toxic, and Renee insisted that I encourage Suzy to break it off, as it was impacting her nerves. He would call her every few minutes to problem-solve, and she was buckling under the stress of it. Fortunately, Suzy understood, and she was able to explain to Richard that he needed to move along.

When the answering machine picked up a call at Suzy's house, you would never get the curt message "Not here; leave a message." You would feel the human warmth on the other end of the phone, her embrace of the caller with her characteristic optimism. Her greeting made you feel that she cared if you had a good day. I loved calling the house because even if I didn't get Suzy, I got this loving hug from the voice on the machine, redefining the phrase, "You had me at hello." Love was always in her voice.

During the time that Suzy lived at the house, she used Access Link, a transport service for seniors and people with disabilities. She learned to schedule her own rides and was such a frequent user that all the drivers knew her well and loved seeing her. She would get on the van and greet them by name with enthusiasm, asking them how their day was going, sometimes bringing them a soda. These people were doing a job in which they were essentially invisible, so the response to her was extraordinary.

Suzy became friendly with some of the seniors using the same route, jumping off the bus to help them with their wheelchairs and doing up their seat belts. I can't say if she was more of a menace than a help, but she got much joy out of being a ray of sunshine. One friend in particular was a senior named Sylvia. "Mommy, Sylvia was so happy to see me on the bus today. She has arthritis in her fingers, so I helped her button her coat, and put on her hat. I told her to stay warm; it's freezing out today." She took pride in helping people, and although Sylvia's coat might have been buttoned completely incorrectly, Suzy felt she was making a difference. "Mommy, Sylvia has invited me to tea at her house."

"Where does she live?" I asked.

"I don't know," she replied, innocently oblivious to the logistical facts. "But I'll go with Access Link, and you can come and pick me up afterwards."

One day, I went on the transportation with Suzy, and I said to Sylvia, "I hope Suzy doesn't bother you."

She replied, "You have no idea what it means to me when I see her on the van. With a son in Colorado and a daughter in New York, Suzy's energy gives me oxygen to breathe. She is such a sweetheart."

I shyly asked again, "But does she really offer you assistance, or is she in the way?"

"No," she answered firmly. "We help each other, and we both feel good about it. It's not always the way it should be. But it's the way it makes us feel that we cherish."

I thought back to the times that Suzy would accompany me to visit my mother in the assisted living facility. The seniors would light up when she walked in. She had the patience of a saint. They would regale her with the same stories over and over again. I was busy looking at my watch, and she would be saying, "Charlie, I know just how you feel."

"When are you coming back?" they would say. The next time she walked in, they would each try to pull her into a conversation with them. "Charlotte, how is your granddaughter? Did she hear from college yet?" She knew everyone's business, and they loved that she showed such an interest in them. "Sylvia, did you remember to take your vitamin C today?" After Sylvia admitted that she forgot, Suzy would say, "Just give me your phone number, and I'll call you every day to remind you. And if you need me to come with you to your appointments at the doctor, I know just how to handle them. You have to advocate for yourself." Her voice could be heard singing through the halls of the nursing home, bringing happiness and friendship to many lonely geriatrics. They asked her to pull the numbers at bingo; even when she was feeling very ill, she did not want to disappoint and would go anyway. One of the seniors asked her if she might like to play, and she answered, "No, thanks, Billy. I get too much pleasure watching you all have fun." That was Suzy's gift. What she lacked in intellect, she made up for in heart.

Suzy was an ambassador for people with developmental disabilities and a living example of a person who against all odds lived a quality life. She was never held back by what medical people would identify as limitations.

Suzy had met another suitor named David and begun a relationship with him. I have never really been able to adequately define the true meaning of love, but as I watched Suzy and David together, they exemplified what I believe it should look like in the purest form. They didn't send out the kind of scent that made one feel they could not wait to be alone. Quite the contrary—they welcomed family and friends to provide company and conversation in which they joyfully participated. They didn't hug or kiss, but they cared for each other in the most basic way. They worried that there was enough food to eat, appropriate clothing to wear, activities to fill lonely moments, and called to make sure they were safe and secure. Suzy was like another mother. She was always guiding him and telling him what to do. When he was invited to someone's home for dinner, she instructed him, "Don't forget to bring a box of candy."

11

I'm Standing with You

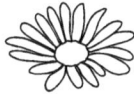

I was July 2013, and Suzy had been living at the Fischer House for nine years. She had suffered through many health crises, and her creatinine levels had risen once more. A twenty-four-hour urine test told us how much urine the body was excreting and the subsequent level of toxins that were building up.

Knowing after the first transplant that she would most likely need a second, the vascular surgeon had chosen to leave the original fistula in her arm. The site of the wound had grown redder and more invasive with each year. Because dialysis was a possibility, we went back to the vascular doctor to check the accessibility of the fistula and confirm that the arteries were all still correctly attached.

The kidney from the first transplant had shriveled to the size of a raisin and lost functionality. We were despondent, desperate, and determined—all three emotions enveloping us relentlessly throughout the day. Suzy was exhausted once again, although still maintaining her ability to function. She barely complained, soldiering on while her body waged a war. Although she was feel-

ing awful, she wanted to work at the summer camp sponsored by
the nursery school where she worked. Yet I saw in her eyes and
her complexion that she was becoming weaker and less able to
muster the strength required to stay on schedule.

Suzy had been on the inactive transplant list for some years,
but at this point, with her dire levels, she crossed over from the
inactive to the active list. She was now eligible, but if we didn't
find a donor soon, she was going to have to go back on dialysis.

I had gone to bed that night with little resistance to my
foreboding thoughts. I knew Suzy would not be able to survive another round of dialysis. It had nearly killed her the first
time. As I prepared for bed, I looked at myself in the mirror,
noticing how the years of neglect had left me with bloat around
my stomach, lifeless hair, and downcast eyes. But the mirror
couldn't see the damage to my essence. The multiple traumas
and stress-filled situations, the worry, and the fear had stripped
me of joy and tranquility. Even so, I never gave in to my mental
fatigue, propelled by the constant love I felt to overcome and
win the battles.

A psychologist I trusted had told me multiple times to stop
questioning God, but I was unable to. I believed there were two
Gods—one good and one evil. Suzy was their prize. The good
God was trying to keep her safe, while the bad God was trying
to destroy her. As her sword and shield, I would fight by her side
until my last breath.

I did not want sympathy or pity. If anyone wanted to express
compassion, I directed them to give it to Suzy. She deserved it
more than I did. Was I flagellating myself for having the cruel
gene that caused her suffering? Maybe, so I pushed myself every
day through each health crisis without ever looking at what my
own life had been. This was my karma, and I wore it like a general.

Remembering to floss my teeth the way the oral hygienist had shown me the week before, I heard the phone next to my bed ringing. It was late, around 11 p.m. There was surely only one reason I was receiving a call at this hour: something was wrong with one of the kids. With enormous trepidation, I ran to pick up the receiver, my head already under a turbulent wave of panic.

"Mrs. Fischer, Jane Fischer?"

I immediately recognized the gravity of the call. I felt my knees warp as my body sagged onto the bed. "Yes, this is Jane. Who is calling?"

"Mrs. Fischer, this is the transplant unit at Saint Barnabas. You must bring Suzy immediately. We have a donor kidney for her."

Was I crying with relief or shock? I screamed for Al, who was unable to sleep and watching a rerun of the game show *Jeopardy*. "Al, come upstairs. It's the hospital. They have a match."

Al came leaping up to the bedroom, took the phone from me and started to ask the practical questions I was too excited to remember. "Whose kidney? How did he die? How old was he? How much time do we have?" When we learned the young man had died of a motorcycle accident at the age of twenty-three, we were sad but most grateful for his bequest.

We went round to get Suzy, who sobbed with survivors' guilt about the young man's fate. "But, Mommy, why did he have to die?" I can't take his kidney. He was so young. He had his whole life in front of him."

I consoled her as best as I could, but it was not easy to convince her that she needed to accept this kidney as perhaps her last hope. "Suzy, it is very sad to think that he died so young. If he were part of our family, we would be grief-stricken. Let us think instead that he did not die in vain. His loss of life will save yours.

You will always be grateful to him and his family. We might never learn their identity, but we will send them a letter anyway, offering our condolences and thanking them for their selflessness."

Suzy seemed to accept my sentiments and went off to get dressed.

Al was waiting in the car when we walked out with her packed bag filled with items for a lengthy stay in the hospital. I had had no time to pack mine, knowing that each minute was critical to the success of the transplant. I was in such a hurry to leave the house that I hadn't noticed one foot was wearing a white Converse sneaker and another a turquoise Nike. I walked unevenly as I helped Suzy to the car. I admonished myself for my carelessness, but it seemed trivial to even mention it on the drive over. Suzy had started to weep again while considering her donor's untimely death.

Arriving at the hospital, I allowed myself a small measure of encouragement. We might have a solution to one of Suzy's problems. Al gave the keys to the valet, and we rushed inside to the intake desk, where the nurse boomed out, "You must be Suzy Fischer. We have been waiting for you to arrive. Mom, please sign this form and we will show you upstairs to the room."

As I scribbled my name, they put Suzy into a wheelchair, and Al carried her belongings. Someone had called the elevator already. We arrived swiftly on the fifth floor, where another team was waiting to put Suzy onto a gurney and begin the testing necessary before the surgery. Al and I put on scrubs, facemasks, and hair bonnets. It felt like a well-rehearsed military operation. If I was in any doubt about the time sensitivity of our decision to accept the kidney, I now became acutely aware of the need for haste as the nursing staff executed precision orders. The young man was being kept alive until the doctors could simultaneously remove and transplant. Although the ideal time for a successful transplant is twenty-four hours, the success of the procedure incrementally improves with each hour less. The nurses were fussing around Suzy, inserting needles, hooking up IVs, checking her temperature, and taking her blood pressure. "Mommy, mommy, I can't see you. Are you here?"

"Of course I am, Suzy. I will be here all the time. I will never leave you alone in the hospital. Dad is going to go and collect some clothes and toiletries for me and an extra pillow."

Then the unthinkable happened. Someone came to tell us that there were no operating rooms available. We would have to wait.

"Wait!" I shrieked. "There is no more waiting we can do."

"Calm down, Jane," Al said, reaching for my hand. "You cannot let Suzy take in your tension. She must remain positive."

So we sat. We drank cup after cup of coffee; we watched other patients being wheeled around. We saw residents come off duty, hardly able to stand after thirty-six hours in the emergency rooms. We dozed off. We engaged Suzy in banal conversation when she wasn't sleeping. But we never saw our surgeons. I was becoming crazy.

After an hour or two, one of the nurses came over, having recognized us from our previous experience on this floor. "Mrs. Fischer, how are you? I am Azalea. I was the nurse on duty when Suzy was here for her first transplant. I remember her incredible spirit during that procedure. She made me love my work and has always remained my favorite patient. I am praying for her today with all my heart. I will be watching over her." I lovingly reached out to Azalea and then gratefully watched as they wheeled Suzy into the operating room where she waved to the team and said, "I'm back!"

I waved at her, but she was dozy from the preanesthetic and couldn't keep her eyes open. I felt a yearning to keep her safe as well as an obligation to trust the doctors. I practiced a belief in a higher power that would bring her back to me with her new kidney, ready to tackle the next phase of her life.

When the surgeons came to tell us that everything had gone according to plan, I was relieved, although still extremely anxious. Al didn't appear to be as distressed as I was, so I deferred to his line of questioning with regard to Suzy's condition. We had been waiting quietly in the corridor for many hours during the surgery, so I blamed my nervousness on my overtiredness. The doctor who spoke was factual, straightforward, and direct. I supposed he was also bone-tired but wished he could find a little more patience as he described the complexity of the surgery. Despite the issues, he felt that the transplant had gone "well." She was making urine, "liquid gold," which was the best sign of a successful transplant. But time alone would demonstrate whether this was the case.

Suzy was currently in recovery, and it was several more hours before we could see her. I paced up and down, impatient to see my girl. I couldn't concentrate on reading, I had nothing to say to anyone, I was thirsty and anxious. We had been joined in the hospital by Ben and Beth, and the four of us glumly stared at one another. Finally, a nurse came to advise us we could go up to the recovery room, as Suzy was waiting to see us.

The room was small, and because Suzy had a roommate, we had to take turns going in. I was the first. With so many needles and tubes and pipes attached to every orifice, I expected Suzy to be in pain and discomfort. She probably was in terrible pain, but she still managed to smile at me and in a hoarse voice say, "Mom, are you OK? I am fine. Please don't worry about me. I need to know how you are."

I assured her I was great, relieved to see she was awake and feeling well enough to channel her thoughtfulness to everyone else's well-being before her own. When one of her favorite nurses came over to check on her, she said to her, "Roz, when can we boogie?" knowing that was this nurse's favorite hobby.

Roz was thrilled to see Suzy. "Not today, Suzy; you must not move. You have weights on your body to keep you still. I'll tell you when it's time."

I have struggled to convey the empathy that is the core of Suzy. She has always been able to anticipate other people's feelings with pinpoint accuracy. With the limitations of Suzy's cognition, it seemed inexplicable that she was able to understand when people were suffering. It confounded everyone who encountered her. She always knew the right words to say, and she said them with earnestness. With her uncanny sensitivity, she melted many icy hearts, and she encouraged reciprocal kindness. I believe that Suzy developed her cognitive empathic skills when she was just a small child. I knew some must surely have been learned in response to what I offered her, but could some have been a result of changes in the OXTR and BDNF genes? We never tested for those genes, but I never stopped being in awe of her pure goodness.

The others were knocking on the door to get their turn to see Suzy. I explained to her that I had to leave for a little while so that Ben and Beth could come in without overwhelming her. Neither Ben nor Beth could see how I was going to sleep on the lounge chair in the room. Since I suffer from chronic stenosis, it wasn't an ideal setup. It did not recline more than 40 percent, it was narrow, and it wasn't cozy.

The next day, Ben came back to the hospital, "smuggling" in an air mattress that we inflated in the room with a pump. It appeared to have a slow hole: over my time in the hospital, I must have blown it up at least three times a day, and it never felt firm. I would begin the night with a relatively solid base beneath my back, but by the morning, I was enveloped in the folded sides, feeling the floor beneath me as the air continued hissing from the invisible escape route. I had to pick up the defective blob of plastic each morning by 7 a.m. and lay it against the window side of the room, allowing the staff some room to walk around the bed.

I was now sixty-four years old, and without constant attention to the strengthening exercises I had been prescribed, I suffered from sciatica. Although I refused to take necessary pain medication, bounding from the chair to the floor took its toll.

Suzy meanwhile remained hooked up to her tubes and lay miserably in the bed. We had learned to navigate the bathroom runs. I would help her from the bed, one arm lifting her weakened body, another holding the roller with the IV. She would gingerly roll out of the bed, careful not to dislodge the catheter or trip over the wires.

We would slowly make our way about the little room. Although there could not have been more than four feet from the foot of the bed to the bathroom door, it would often take us seven minutes. This was sometimes unfortunate, and there were a few occasions when we failed to make the toilet bowl in time. Laughter was the only recourse we had when Suzy watched me on all fours, picking up fecal matter with a garbage bag while holding her IV still with one hand. All credit to Al, when during one of these moments, he was faced with having to clean the bathroom floor. He rose to the occasion with dignity and aplomb, and he learned there was nothing he would not do for his child.

It was vital during this time to keep Suzy immunosuppressed. The risk of infection was high, and each time we came into the room, we would have to cover ourselves from head to toe. The incision area was large and predictably sensitive. The surgeon had made a second cut on the other side of her stomach. Suzy winced when the nurses changed her dressings, but she said nothing. She always introduced herself to a nurse she had never seen before, or greeted a familiar face by her name, asking after her family. The nurses seemed to brighten up upon entering Suzy's room and lingered a little longer than they should have, absorbing some of her light to get them through a difficult day.

On day four after the surgery, a nurse previously unfamiliar with Suzy came in with a somber attitude. She forgot to say hello or enquire as to Suzy's pain levels, so Suzy simply said, "Hello, I haven't seen you here before. My name is Suzy, although you probably knew that from reading my chart. How are you doing? I like your shoes." The nurse looked over at me, not sure how to respond to such sweetness.

When we got the green light to go home, Ben and Beth prepared our house with many welcome home messages and gifts. They filled the refrigerator with fruit and vegetables, low-sodium cold cuts, and healthy snacks. There were flowers in every room, color-coordinated to match the furnishings. They strung banners across the front door and tied bunches of balloons to the door handle. Our homecoming was festive, slightly mitigating the anticipation of isolating ourselves alone at home, which we knew was to follow. We had to keep up a strict vigilance about restricting germs from entering the house.

The doctors were very pleased with Suzy's creatinine levels, and in general the transplant was considered a success. With Suzy seated in the dining room and the family in the living room, we celebrated our good fortune. Prematurely, as it so happened. We were soon plagued by life-threatening ill health.

Suzy had to stay home for four months after this transplant. How she missed living at Fischer House and her social life at Jespy! It was difficult to keep her occupied, especially since she was feeling well and wanted to return to her schedule. We knew at this point that although Suzy's body had accepted this new kidney, there was reflux in both transplanted organs. The first kidney, which was shriveled and virtually inactive, still produced a little urine, which was backing up into the bladder. The second kidney was operating well and producing larger amounts of urine, but this too was backing up into the bladder. The surgeons strongly debated about whether to operate.

As we approached month three of the isolation, the bladder issues began, causing severe spasms and pain. Several consulting doctors had expressed a concern that the reflux was causing the chronic urinary tract infection (UTI), while others felt there was no correlation. There was some speculation that removing the first kidney transplant and then doing a revision of the ureters on the second might ameliorate the reflux. The transplant urology surgeon strongly objected to doing another surgery for fear of life-threatening ramifications. The nephrologist kept insisting on some course of action: "If we don't do something, she is going to die from these infections."

I went back to the nephrologist surgeon who had placed the kidneys in the body and implored him: "I am a lousy quarterback. I can't get anyone to agree. You must help me here. I can't make the decision, yet the urology doctor is frustrated with me. He is saying he will do it without any guarantees. What do I do? I don't want to send Suzy back to surgery, but I don't want her to succumb to one of these infections either."

As Suzy continued to decline in health, we had to face the reality that she needed more care than was available at the

Fischer House. Although there was twenty-four-hour coverage, it was spread over eight-hour shifts, which meant that there was a revolving door of aides that came in and out. We needed one person who would live with Suzy as a companion and have a vested interest in her well-being, not just a watchdog.

We found ourselves having Suzy living at home with us when she felt really sick, but this was psychologically not healthy for her as she resented having to come back to Mommy and Daddy. I had numerous meetings with Jespy, hoping for a different model, but they were unable to meet my requests. I can't blame them, because this was never intended to be a supervised housing situation. Our situation was unprecedented and incompatible with the Jespy model.

One morning we learned about a two-bedroom condo for sale in a building with several Jespy clients. We felt that this might be a better opportunity for Suzy to live with a consistent caregiver. Despite her objections, we tried to convince her why Fischer House wasn't working for her any longer.

Suzy was furious and upset. She felt she was being punished for having all these health problems. She loved the house, she adored her room, and she thrived being the mother hen in the home. This bitter pill presented a very difficult time in her life. When she realized that we were not offering her a choice, she decided to decorate her new flat in the same purple she had chosen for the house and accept that we were providing the best situation for her needs.

Saying goodbye to her roommates was traumatic, and it was compounded when Diane moved into the master bedroom that Suzy used to inhabit. We were torn, watching Suzy sadly unpack her belongings in the new place. It definitely wasn't as luxurious or cozy as the house, but her new aide was able to stay in the bedroom next to hers and would drive her wherever she needed to go.

After several months, Suzy settled in and came to terms with the condo. We had bought a sleeper couch so she could invite her nieces and nephews for sleepovers, and we stocked the kitchen so she could invite friends for dinner.

Her first dinner party included her niece and nephew, Bailey and Cole, and their mom, Britt, Suzy's sister-in-law through her marriage to Ben, who had become Suzy's go-to person. Britt offered Suzy friendship on a one-to-one level, as well as tenderness when family dynamics were strained. Britt was always able to comfort Suzy and give her encouragement when she most needed it.

Beth's daughters, Sydney and Alyssa, came for dessert and games rounding out the raucous evening. Suddenly the apartment didn't seem too bad, and these wonderful evenings became monthly events.

Finding reliable aides would prove to be difficult. The first lady we hired was Abigail. She told us she was unhappy with the two single beds in her room, and that she would pay for a queen mattress to cover them. She and Suzy went off to the mall to make the purchase. When they got there and realized the mattress would cost $900, Abigail said to Suzy that she didn't have the money. Suzy countered, "It's no problem, Abigail. You can put it on my credit card and pay me back."

A few days later, I made a surprise visit to see Suzy around 7 p.m., and I saw Abigail, Suzy, and an unknown gentleman sitting at the table. "Mom, this is George. He is a friend of Abigail's, and he is having dinner with us." I contemplated the situation with some concern.

The next day I asked Suzy, "Darling, is George there often for dinner?"

"No, Mom, but he is here every morning for breakfast. Abigail says he has nowhere to live at the moment, so he is staying in the flat with us." Needless to say, George and Abigail were asked to leave the apartment that day, and the money for the mattress was never recovered.

We had another caregiver who was rather glamorous. She caused a commotion when she insisted that Suzy have a real boyfriend and a sexual relationship. She told me that Suzy was forty-five years old now and should not be virginal. But it was none of the caregiver's business, and neither Suzy nor her boyfriend were interested in an intimate relationship.

Needing a break, Al and I took at trip down to Florida. We had just arrived when I got a call from Renee at eleven in the morning. She had received a call from Suzy's house mother telling her that Suzy had awoken in the middle of the night, panicking that there was a man in her room who was coming to get her. My daughter, Beth, my brother, Neal, and his wife, Judy rushed over to be with Suzy, but when I tried calling her, she screamed at me, saying her mother was dead. I reassured her that it was I on the phone, but she was inconsolable. Al was making flight plans for us to get back to New Jersey.

When we arrived at the airport, I rushed to Beth's house where Suzy was staying, but she refused to recognize me. "Get away from me. My mother is dead. I don't know you. Leave me alone." She was ranting about the ghosts that were coming to get her, and to this day she has a vivid recollection of the images she saw.

Then she would say, "Mommy, get out, get out! They're gonna kill you! Get out!"

I said, "Suzy, honey, it's OK." Finally I said, "It's a nice robber; it's OK." I'd try to go with her into her world, but she was extremely agitated and frightened. "Take me away! Take me away before they kill you! I'm bad, Mommy, I'm bad!"

I brought Suzy to our house thinking the familiarity of her bedroom might snap her back, but she continued to scream through the night. I tried everything to calm her. "Listen, I know you see it, but trust me, it's not real."

That would make her even more angry, because they were real in her mind. "Shut the door, Mommy!"

"Suzy, honey, there's no one there."

"They're there!"

We were afraid, so we locked the door to keep her from harming herself. I pretended to be a friend of her mother's who was going to help her to overcome whatever felt threatening.

By the morning, we were in the emergency room. Suzy was admitted to Saint Barnabas and after a few days transferred to Mount Sinai, where they did a battery of tests that uncovered nothing. Since neither of these hospitals had psychiatric facilities, my nephew, Dr. Ben Yudkoff, who was a psychologist at Harvard, introduced us to a doctor who was an expert in psychosis.

This dark moment, which lasted ten days, was like no other. I didn't know if she could come back from it. We changed her medications to a cocktail that would sedate and calm her fury. My brother weighed in with the thought that her brain was aging and maybe she was starting to experience dementia. I put that thought into a dark cave and walked into the sunlight. I would not let my fears go there.

As the medications continued to allay the tempestuous situation, we were allowed to bring her home, but after a couple days, she started seeing the ghosts again. "Please don't go out. They are going to kill you." She was in a complete state of terror. They had taken over her mind, but I would not allow them to place her in a psychiatric hospital. The doctors gave her a combination of Risperdal and Lexapro, which helped to calm her down.

Suzy went through a complete psychotic breakdown. This was probably the worst of the worst of times I have seen her through. We had daily visits with psychiatrists to ascertain the cause, but it remained a mystery.

12

OOH CHILD

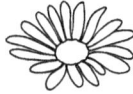

One year at Thanksgiving, one of the grandchildren asked Al and me how we had met. "Oh, now that is a long time ago. We were both studying at Adelphi University in Garden City," I answered.

Al said, "Your grandmother was the most beautiful girl in our graduating class. Everyone wanted to go out with her." Beth looked at me and said, "Mom, tell us the story."

So I began: "Al was handsome, and the president of our class. He was the captain of the baseball team and a phenomenal player. After a couple of dates, we became pinned. That meant I wore his fraternity pin as a symbol of his affection and fidelity and to show everyone we were going steady.

"He was a wonderful boyfriend, so attentive and caring. I was a picky eater, and he always knew how to get me to eat. He didn't pay much heed to his studies, while I was the opposite and always in the library. He wanted to be around me, so he had to come study in the library too, and that semester we both made the dean's list. Your father would have walked on hot coals for me!

"He was the class president, and I was running for class sweetheart. It was a bit silly, I know, but that's what we did in the sixties. There was a tie between a girl called Linda and me. Only the president of the class could cast the deciding vote. Al cast his vote for the other girl. I was devastated. His fraternity brothers told me to break up with him, my brothers were furious, and my parents were upset. I gave him back his pin, and I didn't speak to him for a few weeks."

Al had been sitting quietly waiting for me to finish the story and now piped in. "I still stand behind my decision. I could not let Mommy win based on my vote when we were boyfriend and girlfriend. That was not the honorable thing to do."

After I shunned him for a little while, one of his roommates called me and told me he was suffering enormously. He had been drinking every night and cursing and railing. He begged me to take him back. "Jane, you have punished him enough. He is a wreck."

In our time off, Al had been dating a very pretty girl, and I had been dating a very boring man. I decided I wanted Al back. I went over to his dorm and waited and waited. I had to leave at 11 p.m. as we had curfews back then. I was disappointed, but Al had not yet returned to his dorm.

"Exactly right," said Al. "Your mother came looking for me. She waited all night, but I was out on a date." He was smiling as he told this part. "Well, anyway, I knew she was the girl for me, so I went and threw rocks at her window until she looked down, saw it was me, and told me she loved me."

The family was hanging on every word, laughing at the image of Al throwing rocks to wake me up. I continued: "This was the time of the war in Vietnam, and Daddy had a very low lottery number," which meant that he was likely to be drafted. "He wanted to go to law school, but that was not grounds for a deferment. So the dean at the university suggested that he apply to the National Guard, which he did and got accepted.

"Our wedding, which was on June 28, 1970, took place during his basic training and we weren't even sure if he would get a pass to attend. We had been to so much expense and trouble that we even had someone who could stand in for him in case he didn't make it."

Beth and Ben were looking at me with saucer-shaped eyes, never having heard this story before.

Al was doubled over, laughing, remembering the fellow whom he had coopted to be his body double should he be unable to leave. "Wait; the story isn't over," I said. "Al made it to the wedding on a forty-eight-hour pass. Once he returned to duty, I went back to my parents' house. The neighbors were aghast, thinking the marriage must already be over, since I was returning home."

It was one of the most relaxed family gatherings we ever had. I think the children saw a side to us that was youthful and gay. Al and I had a chance to reminisce about the innocent time in our lives when we were little more than teenagers ourselves.

Suzy took on a great deal of responsibility around my relationship with the rest of the family. For example, Al asked me to go with him for a weekend to our apartment in Florida. I stalled, reluctant to leave Suzy, who had been having numerous health issues. Suzy, feeling herself a constant source of aggravation between us, called my dear friend and her psychologist, Linda Halperin. "Aunt Linda, listen to me. You must convince my mom to go to Florida with my dad. You are the only one she will listen to. I don't care what you say to her, what you make up, but she needs to do this for my father. I'll be fine."

Linda replied, "Suzy, you must understand how much Mom worries about you. She just doesn't feel comfortable about leaving you alone. When you are better, she will travel."

"Aunt Linda, I may never be well enough."

This reply stopped Linda from responding. Instead, she called me and said, "Jane, you must do this for Suzy. She feels such a burden. She is insisting you leave next Thursday. Quite frankly, you must do this, because she is becoming buried in guilt. If she becomes mildly sick, Ben and Beth can handle it, and if she requires you, you are a short plane ride away. If for no other reason than her peace of mind, you must do this."

Linda had known Suzy for many years and understood that she would be devastated if I didn't go. Suzy suffered much in her life, but always put her misfortune after others. She was driven to be a guiding light, a forerunner, a catalyst for change. She loved to make people laugh and see them happy. She was never able to fake a feeling or emotion. If a thought was in her head, it was often on her lips, since discretion is not a word she understands. Loyal to a fault, she seems to have a celestial role on earth.

On one of our many visits to the hospital, she stopped the valet attendant. "Joe, how is your toe?" He helped her out of the passenger seat and replied, "I went to the podiatry center at the VA hospital just yesterday, as I was in a lot of pain."

"Well, make sure you soak it. Put a little salt in the water too," she advised him.

"That's a great idea, Suzy."

As we were walking into the building, she turned back to him and said with a smile, "Joe, think about me getting my own parking spot since I am here so often." Joe smiled at her and promised to keep our car up front.

As we walked into the ward, Suzy stopped to tell a nurse how lovely she looked that day and what a beautiful outfit she was wearing. The nurse was overweight and wearing her scrubs!

Back in 2002, Suzy had begun to suffer from crippling headaches. Since I had always experienced intense migraine symptoms, we felt that it might be hereditary. When they did not abate, we made an appointment with a neurologist, who suggested that we schedule Suzy for an MRI to rule out the possibility of a brain tumor.

When the results came back to us, we were relieved to learn there was no tumor. We knew there was damage in the occipital lobe, and we knew that there was damage in the cerebellar vermis, but we didn't understand a very strong image of something that could be described as a molar tooth at the front of her scan.

Many years later, my brother Marc called me with revolutionary news. He had been reading about the recent discovery of Joubert syndrome, and everything that Suzy had experienced thus far in her life seemed to be consonant with it. Her issues around ocular apraxia, language and speech skills, balance, compromised brain abilities, and organ failure were listed as characteristics of the syndrome. Additionally, the pronounced image of the "molar" in the brain, which we had seen in Suzy's MRI scans, was the definitive marker for the diagnosis.

Joubert syndrome is a genetic disorder that is typically inherited in an autosomal recessive manner. This means that a child must inherit two copies of the defective gene, one from each parent, to develop the syndrome. The syndrome was named after a French pediatrician, Marie Joubert, who first reported on it in 1969. It wasn't until the late 1990s that researchers identified mutations in several genes that were associated with Joubert syndrome, allowing for more accurate diagnosis and understanding of the condition's inheritance patterns.

Al, Suzy, and I were immediately asked to go down to the hospital in Philadelphia, where we were given genetic tests that we had never had before. We were flabbergasted when the results came back. We all carried the gene! The possibility of this was preposterously low.

The entire family was summoned for genetic testing. Fortunately, although some of the family did carry the gene, their partners did not, and the risk of giving birth to a sick child was mitigated.

Since Joubert syndrome has remained a very rare condition, it is not automatically included in the panel of genetic testing that is done before a couple wishes to have a child. I thought back to the decision surrounding Ben's conception. At the time, we were told that there was no evidence to support any chance of having another child with neurological problems. In retrospect, we were very lucky to conceive our beautiful, healthy, perfect Ben, for it could have been a very different story.

I immediately joined the Joubert Syndrome Organization. Suzy appeared to be one of the oldest living people with Joubert's. I was asked to attend the conference in Baltimore the following year, where I would address the concerns of the families.

I wasn't sure what I was going to say to these parents. They were from all over the world, and their children were mostly significantly younger than Suzy. I called home, and Suzy picked up telling me to go out there and "break a leg," a stage term we used when we wanted to encourage one another to excel. "Mom, you can do this. I believe in you." I laughed as she mimicked the words she had heard from me all her life.

Standing in front of these hopeful-looking mothers and fathers, I decided not to read my notes and to ad lib instead.

I truthfully and accurately described what life was like with Suzy and how I had started infant stimulation almost the minute she was born. I went on to explain how her independence was largely motivated by her confidence, which I had spent years honing. I stressed how important it was to keep teaching, encouraging and above all loving these children. I had no blueprint to offer, no hard-and-fast rules, just suggestions that had worked for our family.

Many individuals approached me during the conference to ask me about what would happen to their children. I did my best to answer, but although Suzy had risen above her disabilities, I could not say that another child would.

One grandmother had come along to help babysit another child in the family, and she was brimming with questions for me. My best advice for her was to accept the diagnosis of the doctors and not to imagine it was less serious than she was told. I asked her to give love and patience to the entire family, as it would become a family affair. No one would be exempt from the demanding schedule of a child with special needs.

Although we had been given a name for Suzy's condition, it did not alter her life in any way. I was even grateful that I had never known about it, as I would most likely have been waiting for an organ to fail and worrying long before it was necessary. Nothing changed in our routines, and we simply kept moving forward in the best way possible.

One of the most important ingredients to quality of life for Suzy was her job at Temple B'nai Jeshurun, in Short Hills, New Jersey. Back in 2001, Barbara Hochberg, who was the director of the preschool at that time, had adopted a philosophy around accepting children with special needs even though they were not a special education facility. She wanted to allow every child and their family the opportunity to be part of their school community.

With this open-minded approach, I felt that Suzy could be a wonderful asset to the early childhood program as a classroom assistant and called Barbara to ask whether she would entertain the thought. After I described Suzy's achievements as well as her difficulties, Barbara explained that Suzy would have to provide a résumé and interview for the position just like anyone else.

Suzy made the appointment and went to see Barbara, who called me after their meeting to tell me the news: "I have been interviewing applicants for many years, some good, some bad. Suzy blew me away. She probably was the best interviewee I ever had. She was smartly dressed and had all her information (including references) with her. She let me know exactly what her strengths were and how valuable she would be to my staff."

Barbara hired her and she has been with the school for twenty-three years. Barbara was succeeded by Michelle Feingold, who also admires and respects Suzy and has shown tremendous support through the years with her friendship and love.

One day Suzy said to me, "Mom, I have been working at B'nai Jeshurun for fifteen years. How come they have never given me a raise?" I chuckled lightly and went to see the director of the school, asking her to add an extra $100 to Suzy's salary, which I had been secretly paying since her first day. The next week, Suzy came home excitedly, exclaiming that they must have read her mind, for she received her increase in salary!

Suzy touched the hearts of not just the students but the teaching staff as well. Every year in February, the parents made an elegant luncheon to honor the eighty-plus members of staff. There were usually ten to twelve tables set up. When Suzy entered the room, teachers from every table jumped up and yelled, "Suzy, here! We saved you a seat." Suzy had to table-hop so as not to hurt anyone's feelings.

Suzy became an invaluable member of the school, always remembering items other teachers would forget, always willing to work on hot, humid days during summer camp in the sun, always wearing a cheerful disposition despite her physical pain.

The most significant observation about Suzy came from the rabbi himself: "Jane, every Friday night I try to teach people a little something. By discussing moral principles, I hope to foster a sense of learning and growth within the congregation. Looking around the sanctuary, I notice some people listening, some on their phones, and others distracted and uninterested. And then I try to understand why it is that when Suzy walks into school in the morning, she is able to impart valuable lessons just by her presence. She doesn't have to prepare a sermon or present a topic. She simply *is*. And her *is* is created by embodying her authentic best every day."

Unfortunately, with so many illnesses, Suzy has had to miss many days of work, and I heard from the teachers that the children would all be anxiously waiting for "Miss Suzy" to return. She lit up the classroom with her beautiful smile. For her part, Suzy has always proclaimed that no prescription medicine has been able to heal her better than the love she has received from the staff at B'nai Jeshurun.

13

I'M A SURVIVOR

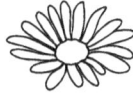

Then we arrived at a crisis point. It was November of 2022. We were celebrating Thanksgiving with all the family. I was hosting at our home, with Suzy acting as my sous-chef and cohostess. She hand-made the decorations for the table and had chosen the place settings. She had suggested that everyone come in color-coordinated shades of orange and brown and sent links to Amazon sites where her nieces and nephews could find sweaters and leggings.

Since Suzy wasn't feeling well, she had slept at home the night before. Early that day, she warned me that she was sure her fever was rising. She made me promise not to say anything because she didn't want to be responsible for canceling this beautiful holiday lunch. Jola, Suzy's companion, helped us to serve the first course, which was a beautiful deep orange pumpkin soup. I glanced over to see Suzy unable to lift her spoon to her lips but refrained from pointing it out to the others. We brought out the second course: the turkey, the stuffing, cranberry sauce, and all the sides. Suzy had left the table and gone over to the sofa to lie down. I couldn't ignore this any longer, so I took her temperature and panicked. It was 104°F. Should we call the ambulance or take her ourselves? Knowing that if we called the ambulance, she would be admitted faster, we dialed 911 and waited just ten minutes for them to come. Meanwhile, I packed a few things for her. I instructed everyone else to finish their meal together, and I would keep them posted once we had some news to share.

The emergency crew came into the house. When they approached Suzy, she weakly lifted herself and offered them some turkey and trimmings. She also apologized for calling them away from their families. The four large men strapped her in, lifted her onto the gurney, and off we went. I sat in the back of the ambulance as the siren screeched through the quiet holiday streets.

The skeleton staff at the hospital, recognizing us, hurriedly ushered us up to a ward. By now Suzy was falling in and out of sleep. She was hooked up to IVs in a matter of minutes to hydrate her body with a saline solution. Suzy, vulnerable and helpless, was drooling from her open mouth and burning up. Doctors and nurses surrounded us, and within hours, it was determined that she had a superbug that was resistant to most antibiotics. The only drug that might be effective, ertapenem, would be most powerful if applied intravenously.

I was scared. Her life hung in the balance. Superbugs are highly contagious and passed not through respiratory contact but through skin to skin contact. My hair was in a cap, booties on my feet, and a long gown covered my body. I washed my hands incessantly.

For twenty-four hours, the situation could have gone anywhere. The family had cleaned up the house and made their way over to the hospital. They were waiting in the corridor for some news. I texted Al with an update, and we waited. And we waited. I urged everyone to go home and get some rest, and I would call with news when I had some. I never took my eyes off Suzy. I knew we were at the end of the line here. She didn't respond to any conversation. She didn't eat. She didn't even wake up most of the time. The doctors came in and out of the room shaking their heads, looking past my enquiring eyes with pessimistic grimaces.

Then on Sunday, three days after starting the medicine, her fever declined to acceptable levels. Suzy opened her eyes and saw me sitting close to her with worry etched all over my face. "Mom, where am I?" I rang the bell for the nurse, trying to hold back the tears until I could stand up and go to the bathroom so Suzy wouldn't feel my worry. "Mom, are you OK?"

My child was asking *me* if I was OK? "If you knew Suzy like I knew Suzy"—those are the only words that came to mind.

Suzy was in the hospital for nine days in a completely sterile ward, followed by six weeks of daily infusions of the antibiotic. For approximately three hours each day, we sat in the oncology department, a needle inserted into her vein. These were long, boring hours when we were too distracted to watch television, read, or concentrate on a conversation. Suzy would doze off, but when a nurse would come in, she always complimented them on their outfit or their shoes. Her sepsis was abating, but the side effects from the drug were debilitating. She suffered terrible bouts of diarrhea and had to wear diapers in case of accidents. Her stomach ached. She had ringing in her ears. We feared that she had C. diff, an infection that results from destroying all the healthy bacteria in the body. We tested her stool and cheered when the culture came back negative. She was allowed to take imodium for the diarrhea, which seemed to help a little.

Then her liver functions took a dive. This could have been a result of the ESBL (superbug) infection or the strength of the antibiotics. Every time we went in, they would run new tests, and by now, all her levels were off. So, they decided to cut back on the Myfordic, the immunosuppressant drug she had been taking for years, in the hope that she would develop some anti-bodies of her own.

I was grateful for the assistance of Lisa Jasinski, whom we had originally met when she managed various homes for Jespy. When she retired from Jespy, we were able to hire her part-time, and she is the only person Suzy would consider as a suitable replacement for me. When Lisa was with Suzy, I was able to rest, confident that Suzy would receive the same loving attention I showered her with. Lisa has remained in our lives both professionally and as a beloved member of our inner circle.

We were living on the edge. The risk versus benefits at stake were enormous. If they cut back on the immunosuppressant drugs, she could reject the kidney. But she could also die from what was happening in her body, because she had no immune system. I was silently hysterical, not knowing which direction was the right one. The doctors were constantly in and out of her room, but they too were at their wits' end. I was frustrated with some of them because of a lack of communication between them. The nephrologists, Dr. Ryan Goldberg and Dr. Luigi Bonomini, were frantically looking for solutions for Suzy while managing my panic. They cared a great deal about her but were not sure about the next course of action.

When we finally finished the treatment, it was time for Suzy to go back into the hospital to do ureter surgery for the reflux. It had been scheduled for January 5, 2023. With only two days of respite from the end of the first ertapenem, she was put on the next dose, this time as a prevention. The doctors had agreed that they would remove the first kidney and reattach the second one to the ureters in one operation. The risks of this were preferable to the risks of two general anesthetics.

Owing to the amount of scar tissue around the incisions for the kidney transplants (one on the left and one on the right), the surgeons planned to make a third incision down the middle of her stomach for this procedure. Opening a flap to the right, they removed the first nonfunctioning transplanted kidney, and opening the flap to the left, they redid the attachment of the ureter.

After the surgery, we had one more week of back and forth to the chemotherapy ward to continue the antibiotic. Suzy was healing nicely, and I conceded that this may indeed have been the problem.

A day or two after the last dose of ertapenem, Suzy uttered the miracle words we had been waiting to hear for years. "Mommy, I am pain-free." I repeated this over and over: "Pain-free." Nectar, nirvana, bliss. We were loving life, laughing, totally relaxed. It seemed miraculous.

We celebrated amongst the family. We carefully hosted little dinners, anxious for her siblings to spend time with Suzy, but conscious of keeping her in a sanitized atmosphere. We played music and danced with the fervor of a hostage freed from his captives. And indeed Suzy felt liberated. Freed from pain but always in fear that it would return.

The snow fell on the ground, and we huddled under heavy comforters, watching reruns of our favorite movies. I allowed my nerves to relax while reading a book on a chaise longue. I rested while Suzy spent hours on the phone recanting her treatment plan to her friends. Our house was filled with relief and repose, buoyant with hope.

Then one morning two weeks later, as I was finishing my breakfast, I heard Suzy calling for me from upstairs. Her neediness was alarming, her consternation unmistakable. "Mommy . . . mom . . . mom." With each syllable, her voice faded. I climbed the stairs and found her in the bathroom, panties on the floor, tears of frustration and despondency pouring forth. Those sweet eyes pleaded with me to do something. "Mommy, it burns so much."

I wanted to rail at God. What was his plan here? I slumped to the floor where she sat, hugged her to me and without conviction, promised we would find a cure. My body told the story. I lacked the energy to get to my feet, felt short of breath. We sat on the floor for a good while as I alternated between desperation and fury. I was crashing without a safety harness.

By 2:00 p.m. we were back in the hospital, evidence of the ESBL superbug strongly present in the bloodwork. Even the serious urologist, the man who refused to reveal his gentler side, broke his stony mien. "Mrs. Fischer, I am so sorry. We took a calculated risk, and unfortunately we were unable to come out on the right side of the equation." He reached out to me, an uncharacteristic gesture that I appreciated with surprise. The nephrologist, who had believed wholeheartedly that the surgery would give Suzy some relief, was dismayed. His disappointment was evident by his gentle and compassionate approach to Al and me.

The infectious-disease doctor was called in for consultation, and he determined that she should begin a new course of ertapenem. Another six weeks of daily visits to the hospital for the infusions began.

I was speechless, flabbergasted at her diagnosis. Suzy lay listlessly in her bed, hooked up to machines, obediently turning this way and next as the nurse requested. "Forgive me," I muttered under my breath. I felt a great deal of responsibility for her well-being. I was making decisions with a machine-like response, based on the evidence the doctors presented. My trust in experts seemed misguided. They didn't know how to help her. The doctors were stumped, finally admitting that her case was one of the most difficult to treat. I tempered myself, knowing that there might not be a good decision to make.

"Mommy, I've had it. I am tired of doctors. I am tired of tests. I am tired of medicine." Suzy was feeling helpless and hopeless, but within seconds, she rebounded with, "Mom, what is the next solution going to be? I want to feel better and get back to my life."

I always tried to be Suzy's defender and keep her spirits lifted, but I must admit that this time it was impossible. We fell into a funk. We spent the next week in the hospital and then began another round of outpatient visits to the chemotherapy center for the infusions. A couple of the patients who were there for cancer treatment on an ongoing basis recognized us from the previous time. Despite their significant frailties, they encouraged us to keep up our spirits. Men and women without hair, vomiting in buckets, so weak they couldn't stand without help, shared the little strength they had and made the experience less unbearable. Suzy was better tempered than me during these times, and she would sometimes bring in little gifts for her friends with warm and cheerful words of encouragement engraved somewhere.

I woke up every morning, dressed myself in warm sweats, and helped Suzy to pick out some comfortable clothing, and with sandwiches in hand, we drove towards the hospital. I found it hard to concentrate on a book. Sometimes we dozed off. Sometimes we were on our phones.

As we were driving over one day, we heard the words to "Survivor" by Destiny's Child.

We decided that would be our war cry during these times. After a few days of quietly singing the song to each other, we asked the patient next to us to join in. Then the next day he asked the patient on the other side of him to join in, and the following day there was a domino effect, with everyone wanting to sing out loud.

We conspired to organize a sing-along at 10 a.m. every morning. The nurses got wind of our plans, and every morning they would stand just outside the cubbies, joining in for the chorus. It was a galvanizing call to bravery, and there was a palpable shift in energy and humor in the patients. I believe the nurses wanted to continue the practice after we left but couldn't find a cheerleader like Suzy.

For several months Suzy tested negative for ESBL. However, her pain remained at a level 7 or 8 out of 10, and on top of this she developed urge incontinence. This meant that she would suddenly get the overwhelming feeling of needing to pee and if she couldn't make it to the bathroom on time, the urine would leak on the floor. Suzy was much too young to develop this condition, so we headed to see a urogynecologist, who diagnosed her with interstitial cystitis. With this condition, the bladder is irritated and scarred and unable to hold urine. In most people, this is not a painful condition, but in Suzy's case, her bladder had been left inflamed from the many bacteria she had hosted. For five months, she tested negative for infection, yet the pain continued unabated.

Then in August 2023, she was found to be carrying Proteus mirabilis, a bacterium known to cause urinary tract infections (UTIs). We tried not to panic. After all, the doctors had not promised that she would never get another infection again. The pain was growing in intensity, and on the Thursday of that week we went back for another culture. On Sunday morning at 11:00 a.m.,

I received a call from the surgery urologist. "Mrs. Fischer, she has Klebsiella, another bacteria causing urinary tract infections."

I had to think before answering. "Is this cycle starting again? Was the surgery then not a success?" The doctor sounded hesitant when he said, "I have a call scheduled with your infectious disease doctor, Dr. Weiner, and he will decide on a treatment plan."

I had considered whether Suzy had an indelible footprint of pain in her psyche and perhaps she imagined it. Before the doctor called me on Sunday morning, I was beginning to become intolerant. I was short with Suzy, suggesting that perhaps she must learn to live with this pain. How guilty I felt when it was confirmed that she had a terrible infection and her pain was very real.

I had been reconsidering the idea of Western medicine as the only solution to Suzy's ongoing pain, which led me to read about a nurse who had spent years studying UTIs and interstitial cystitis. She believed that just as you can't fix a leaky roof if you only plug one or two holes when there are ten, there is more to breaking the cycle of recurrent UTIs and eliminating embedded infections. To determine the other contributing factors, several additional tests are needed. These include looking at vitamin D levels; reducing ammonia levels, which cause damage to the bladder wall; testing for the genetic issues that make it difficult to break down biofilms; and screening for other factors such as mycotoxins and tick-borne infections.

The doctor would not give us an appointment without a Zoom conversation with one of Suzy's current doctors. This was obviously incredibly difficult to schedule, so we were very grateful when the young transplant nephrologist agreed to take a ninety-minute Zoom meeting, especially since he was Jewish and this was scheduled for Yom Kippur, the holiest day of the Jewish calendar.

When we went into his rooms the following week, I asked him to bill me for the call, but he refused, offering the following reason: "Suzy is the patient that reminds me why I got into the medical field to begin with. Her recovery is of the utmost importance to me, and I would do anything to facilitate the diminishment of her pain and discomfort. She has shown bravery and dignity each time I have met with her."

Suzy leaned forward in her chair. "What do you like to eat, Dr. Goldberg? I would love to take you to dinner, but I know you don't have time. So I am going to get you a gift certificate to a restaurant of your choice."

Both the doctor and I were amazed at this suggestion. This girl, who could not go to the store alone and come back with the right change, was astute enough to recognize that the doctor had been unsparing in his care and concern for her. There was never any rhyme or reason about Suzy's brain function.

I was unable to start Suzy on this alternative course, because no sooner had we cleared the way for her to begin the treatment than she was back in the hospital, this time with ESBL and an upper respiratory infection. She had begun a new round of ertapenem and we were driving to the hospital every day once again, but only for three weeks this time. Her veins were impossible to find, which meant they had to insert a PICC line: a long, soft catheter that is inserted into a vein in the upper arm. This is done using ultrasound and a good deal of lidocane. Through this portal, they could feed the antibiotics.

I had wanted to avoid admitting Suzy to the hospital again and hoped we could just go to the short stay department at the transplant hospital. However, when the nurse examined Suzy and realized how ill she was, we were sent directly to the emergency room and had to spend a couple of nights in a ward.

There was an empty bed next to Suzy's in the room, and my other kids urged me to sleep in it overnight instead of the chair, which didn't recline. Neither Suzy nor I felt comfortable with that decision, but a little later on, I thought I might just take a nap on that bed. Of course, I fell asleep and only woke when the orderly came into the room mistaking me for the patient. He apologized for waking me up, asked me how I was feeling, and took out his thermometer to take my temperature. I embarrassedly confirmed I was the mother of the patient who was in the next bed and that I didn't need his attention.

My brothers had begun to question my judgment on this endless parade of doctors and hospitals. They wanted to prepare me for the inevitable. Each time, I would yell, "But we have to try everything. I am not leaving any stone unturned." They would answer, "For what Jane, for what? One of these bugs is going to kill her."

I knew this. I wasn't in denial. But I was also convinced that Suzy wanted me to keep on finding whatever quality I could for her life. Neither of us were ready to hang up our gloves. As long as we both had breath in our bodies, I was going to keep looking for the answers. If it was a month or a year, my mission was to keep gluing her back together.

Beth dropped by to see us one night and pulled me aside to say "Mom, you look exhausted. You can't continue like this at your age. You are seventy-five years old. Can you please take some time for yourself?"

Al was making sure that I was still coming to Florida, anticipating that I might cancel because of how sick Suzy was. Ben was nagging me: "Mom, you have to go away with Dad. You can leave Suzy with us. She will be fine, and you are only two hours away. You must go."

No one understood that I wasn't ready to give up; nor was Suzy. She was still anxious to return to her apartment at Jespy, and despite the pain, she intended to go back to her job at the nursery school, where the children were anxiously waiting for her to return. She had determined that her pain levels were bearable. I was monitoring the side effects of the medications, ensuring that her diet didn't aggravate the diarrhea. Her spirits were chipper, and I was coping and still hoping to accompany my husband to Florida.

They said I have had no life. The generalization galled me, as *they* were holding me to their standards of what a life should look like. From middle-class suburbia, that means restaurant dates with other couples, annual trips to Europe, and bridge games at the club. They were assuming they knew what made me happy, what fulfilled me.

But Suzy was a miracle. She gave me life. Through her, I became a better version of anything I could ever have been. Through her, I became the recipient of the purest version of love. I have never felt hard done by, never wished for anything other than what I have had. I have been completely fulfilled. I feel that my life was touched by an angel—a Suzy angel who has filled my every pore with her gentle essence. She was never able to fake a feeling. If a thought was in her head, it was often on her lips. Loyal to a fault, she seems to be celestial.

Caring for a disabled child has been challenging and demanding, but it has been filled with much love and many rewards. It was not just my obligation, but also my choice to be Suzy's caregiver and dedicate my life to her. Ensuring her safety and well-being far surpassed any personal ambitions. This has been my destiny, and through Suzy I hope I have helped others.

14

YOU ARE SO BEAUTIFUL TO ME

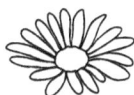

I longed for the quiet of a boring existence and the ability to dream in Technicolor. I knew better than to expect that, so I told myself I would be satisfied just to enjoy a full night's sleep.

My brain was always in an excited state of extrasensitivity, trained after years of trauma to be aware of potential dangers everywhere. This hypervigilance had made me nervous, worried, and anxious. I jumped when there was an unexpected noise, I was filled with fear, and I was overprotective. My acute anxiety often led me down the rabbit hole to depression, but I didn't have the luxury to let that state go on for too long, as I had to be the optimist in the family.

During the early years, Suzy took up most of my time, and Ben and Beth took the rest. I accepted the theory that Al and I, as willing parents, had no right to a life of our own, so I ignored both his and my needs. Al was tough, and I had to become tougher.

Both our mothers had offered support and help, which we relied on tremendously. Their contribution to our lives was enormous and allowed Al to work long hours and me to concentrate on the children. The loss of these two women was devastating.

My two brothers, Neal and Marc, and their respective wives and children, Judy and Mona, Ben, Sunny, and Dari, Aliza, and Shira, made up the village required to raise a child. They reinforced the foundation of our principles, providing additional resources for hope, love, and belonging. Suzy was "Special Aunt Suzy" to the younger members and was invited to be an integral part of all their celebrations in an exalted capacity. I am grateful to all of them for never forgetting to include my special daughter in their simchas (joys) as a bridesmaid, babysitter, and beloved cousin.

Our home had become ground zero for calamities and adversity, but I always tried to add balance to our lives by entertaining, celebrating holidays, and bringing joy wherever possible. Our family moved silently and bravely through the seasons, seizing the good times and bracing for the bad.

Al was resentful, and under my loving façade, I was angry. Our family was broken in many ways but survived each disaster to stand stronger for the next one. We loved one another with fierce loyalty, devotion, and an unhealthy amount of resentment.

Hoping to understand a little about how Suzy related to herself, my co-writer asked me one day if she could interview Suzy. With Suzy's hospitalizations and frequent illnesses, the date kept moving, and when we were finally able to set a date, Suzy had just completed another round of antibiotic infusions to combat a superbug. She was just settling back into her own apartment after living with me and was anxious to get on with her life. This is how the interview, which took place in early 2024, went:

Carol Ann: Suzy, I am so excited to speak to you. I have been waiting quite a long time.

Suzy: Me too. It's good to see you, Carol Ann.

Carol Ann: Suzy, I have some questions for you, but please let me know if any of them make you feel uncomfortable. You can always choose not to answer.

Suzy: OK, no problem.

Carol Ann: Do you see yourself as a person with a disability?

Suzy: Yes, I see myself with a disability. I have motor apraxia. My balance. I have trouble crossing the street. My head goes up and down sometimes. I can't focus when the sun is in my eyes.

Carol Ann: Is that the extent of it, or is there anything else you might like to do that you can't?

Suzy: Mostly things to do with balance. And speech and language.

Carol Ann: Who is the most important person or people in your life, and why?

Suzy: My mom—my mom is my hero. And my brother Ben, because he was my coach when I was doing Tournament of Champions. And Beth, because she played with me and taught me many things. And my nieces and nephew. Dad's good too.

Carol Ann: What would you say about your mom?

Suzy: For forty-nine years, we have had a bond that doesn't go away. She is always with me and by my side. But she annoys me too. She smothers me. I want her to go and enjoy her life. My brother and sister are there: my mother needs to be with my father. She sacrifices too much for me. She slept with me in the hospital; she takes me to the doctors. I'm her life. She needs to take baby steps. She needs to let me go and stop sacrificing for me. Mom, enjoy your life; go do your plans. Let me live mine.

Carol Ann: But if mom wasn't there, who would help you with the doctors and hospitals?

Suzy: I have a companion who can take me. She won't sleep with me in the hospital, but she can do the other things with me. My mom needs her own life.

Carol Ann: What is the key ingredient for you to have quality of life?

Suzy: My health issues. I want to be well. I like to exercise. I have a personal trainer twice a week on Zoom. We do downward dog, balancing exercises, squats, bands, and stretches. I like to go for walks. I like to dance.

Carol Ann: Do you have a favorite hobby?

Suzy: Yes, going on computers. The Internet. I like Facebook and Instagram. I like shopping on the Internet, mostly for my nieces and nephews and my mom. Ninety-nine percent of the time I buy for other people. Very dangerous for me: I have a little bit of a shopping addiction.

Carol Ann: I know you have an amazing memory. What do you remember about your childhood?

Suzy: I remember Panda. They stole Panda. I went to Harrison Middle School and ECLC. I went to Camp Northwood for eight years. My mom's mom used to drive me to school if my mom couldn't do it. I had a lot of therapies. My grandma used to bake me cakes and apple pies. Her second husband used to mail them to me. I remember when my sister went to college, I had a breakdown and asked to go away too. So I went to Maplebrook. I was the treasurer at school. And I was the prom queen.

Carol Ann: What's your best thing to do?

Suzy: Come to my condo and go to my volunteer job.

Carol Ann: What do you hate most about your life?

Suzy: Being sick. All the back and forth. I have just spent weeks of going back and forth to the hospital to have an infusion of antibiotics every day. I just want to be home, living my life. I'm better now.

Carol Ann: What are you looking forward to now that you can stay at home?

Suzy: Spending time with my friends. Making my own arrangements.

Carol Ann: If someone was describing you without having met you, what do you think they would say about you?

Suzy: That I am kind. And sweet. I did more than everyone thought I could. I am playful. Determined. Strong.

Carol Ann: Do you work hard to be that person, or it just flows from you?

Suzy: It is natural for me. When I look at myself in the mirror, I see a kind person with a big smile and a huge heart. I see braveness, kindness, a good heart.

Carol Ann: If you could change something about your appearance, what would that be?

Suzy: My weight. I want to be slimmer. I want to wear a bathing suit and look good in it. I don't want to wear a cover-up.

Carol Ann: Do you like to read?

Suzy: Yes, we have a book club. We are reading romance novels. I like love stories.

Carol Ann: How about TV? What shows do you enjoy?

Suzy: *The Price Is Right. Let's Make a Deal. Chicago MD.* I watch the news. *Grey's Anatomy.* I used to watch soap operas—*General Hospital.*

Carol Ann: Is there anything in life you have missed out on because of your disability?

Suzy: Driving, marriage, and babies.

Carol Ann: And I believe you have a boyfriend?

Suzy: Yes, David. We go for walks together; he is my companion. He is someone in my life. I don't want marriage. Just a boyfriend. I do stuff with him. We go to dinner. But he is annoying, just like all men. We speak most nights.

Carol Ann: Do you have a goal? Is there something you would like to achieve?

Suzy: Yes, I like to go to classes. I signed up for adult education. I'm doing paint-by-numbers and dancing.

Carol Ann: I hear you are an amazing dancer. Do you get the opportunity to dance often?

Suzy: Yes, I dance at the bar mitzvahs of my nieces and nephews. And sometimes we have a dance at Jespy.

Carol Ann: Suzy, how would you tell a stranger to act towards you when they meet you for the first time?

Suzy: I would tell them I have had a disability for forty-nine years, but I don't give up. I would try to make them comfortable by telling them I have problems with balance. I have a disability, but I have the same emotions as everyone else. I cry, I laugh, I am happy, and I am sad. Don't treat me differently. I want you to talk to me as you would talk to someone normal. I would tell them how I feel.

Carol Ann: What makes you the happiest?

Suzy: Being here in my condo at Jespy, where I have the freedom to be me, to be with my friends, to go to my activities. I have support if I need it, but I just want to live my life the way I know how to.

Carol Ann: What makes you the saddest?

Suzy: Sickness. Being home with my mom and dad. Being sick. Feeling bad.

Carol Ann: I know you suffer a lot with debilitating pain. What gives you the strength to get through it?

Suzy: I take one day at a time. I try to keep a positive attitude. I hate going to the doctors and the hospitals, but I know they are trying to keep me well and doing their best. When I am at work or in my condo, I don't even think about it. I am just happy. I have wonderful doctors. Sometimes I am sick, sometimes not. This too shall pass. I don't want to think about it. I go on with my life.

Carol Ann: Do you ever feel embarrassed or ashamed that you are different?

Suzy: No. Not at all. I keep working harder. Sometimes learning is difficult for me. I need to try more. It takes me a long time to learn reading and math and spelling.

Carol Ann: Do you know what EQ is? Does Mom use the expression with you?

Suzy: Yes, mine is off the charts.

Carol Ann: How did that happen?

Suzy: Life. I was born with it. I know how to have compassion and empathy for others. Its natural.

Carol Ann: Do you have a favorite food?

Suzy: Salmon. Salmon with mushrooms. No sauce. In the oven or a frying pan. Plain, grilled.

Carol Ann: You eat out sometimes?

Suzy: Yes, but the food at Jespy is good too.

Carol Ann: Describe your life at Jespy, please.

Suzy: Independent. I go to book club and photography club. I have a lot of friends. We do activities. We watch movies. The food is good. We play Scrabble. We hang out on the weekends.

Carol Ann: Do you have any limitations in life? Is there anything you cannot do?

Suzy: No, I don't think so.

Carol Ann: What frustrates you?

Suzy: I can't drive. Sometimes the computer frustrates me.

Carol Ann: What's your favorite season of the year, and why?

Suzy: Spring and summer, because you can wear short sleeves. I can go for walks outside. I like running. I used to play tennis and ride horseback. I like being active.

Carol Ann: How do you deal with people who are not nice to you? Can you forgive them?

Suzy: I was asked to speak to a group of kids at Mount Pleasant School about my experience of being with girls who did not include me in their group. I had a problem in sixth grade. They were mean to me. I ignored them and went someplace else so they wouldn't bother me.

Carol Ann: How do you remain so kind to people who are not kind to you?

Suzy: I don't know, give them a break. I just wake up and try to find the good in myself and search for the good in people. Just born that way.

Carol Ann: Suzy, do you ever get to the point where you are so sick you just can't take it anymore? Does it occur to you to say, "I can't take this anymore?"

Suzy: Uh-huh. When I was in the hospital now with the super-bug, I said to my mother, "Enough is enough." When they told me I had ESBL again, I started to cry and say, "Oh, no, I can't take any more." But then I pulled myself together. We don't know the cause of it. I find my spirit wherever I go.

Carol Ann: Is there anything in life that you are afraid of?

Suzy: No, no. Nothing worries me.

Carol Ann: Is there anything else you might like to share with me?

Suzy: I have the best family. Wonderful aunts and uncles. Before they moved, I used to work for my Aunt Judy once a month. I went to the Christmas party, the retirement party. My sister's kids give me so much love, like my family in Washington. They know I can't have kids, so they include me in their families. Beth and Ben's kids are wonderful to me. Everyone includes me in the family.

Carol Ann: What would you tell parents who discover they have a child with learning disabilities?

Suzy: Make an appointment with the doctor. Find out what is wrong. Do therapies to help. Give lots of hugs, love, and support. My mom has been my hero. I tell her all the time how much I appreciate what she does for me. Mom, you are my angel. You stay in the hospital with me. You take time off. She is so helpful. She found a doctor on YouTube, and she's taking me for another opinion. She does her homework. I tell her all the time that I appreciate it. Mom, you do everything for me.

Carol Ann: You must hate the doctor visits already.

Suzy: It's enough. Enough already. But this week I only went once. It's a constant. Today I had another urine culture. Next week I have more. I want freedom from the hospital. I want to be with my aide, be with my friends, go to activities, go to my job.

Carol Ann: My last question for you is, what does this book mean to you?

Suzy: I want readers to see what I go through, what I have to do every day. I want to encourage others to keep a positive attitude, to keep fighting. To be strong. Have a routine. Have a purpose in life. Don't think about it. Just be. Don't give up. Some days are good, some days bad. I keep busy, get up in the morning, go to work, go on with my life.

Carol Ann: Thank you so much Suzy. This was a wonderful opportunity to chat with you.

Suzy: Bye, Carol Ann, Thank you. Have a good night.

Did we have a reliance, a codependency, or a dependent codependency? When Suzy was little, I learned that I had to give support to her endeavors to conquer the simplest tasks. This meant helping her to find ways to cope and rebound when she faced a setback.

I was chastised by some very wise teachers when they saw me as coddling her, which was a detriment to her finding independence. I was sending the message that she couldn't care for herself or achieve the tasks before her. I was an enabler. I had to step back and allow her to fall, fail, and finally flourish as she became resilient and confident when her many attempts succeeded.

Enabling is defined as the act of reinforcing behavior that is ultimately unhelpful to your child. Most parents have nothing but good intentions when they inadvertently enable their children. They usually want to protect them from fear, sadness, pain, embarrassment, and failure. Unfortunately, when we prevent our kids from making mistakes and taking risks, we deprive them of important lessons. Kids who never take risks don't learn how to manage risk, and kids who aren't allowed to overcome their errors never learn that messing up isn't the end of the world. I have always told my children that if you make a mistake and learn from it, it is a very valuable lesson.

Suzy is a force who strives to find her own way to live her life most productively, while I wanted to protect Suzy from negative emotions such as fear, sadness, pain, and embarrassment.

When I read the interview she gave to Carol Ann, I realized again how much she yearned for her independence and freedom from me. That interview invited me to examine the dynamics of our relationship. She imitated and repeated conversations that she had overheard between other family members, who constantly suggested I cultivate other interests. She internalized a lot of guilt, because she felt responsible for monopolizing my attention. As a result of these feelings, she gently reminded me I should have some fun with my friends and my husband.

In the early 2020s, with Suzy battling so many health issues, my brothers, Marc and Neal, who had supported me in their medical capacity from the first moment, became extremely concerned about me. They had plied me with critical information and assistance throughout Suzy's life. But as the health conditions became more dire, and the hospital visits more frequent, they begged me to stop running from one specialist to another. They wanted Suzy to enjoy the life she had been given and for me to stop tugging on her, insisting we try one more cure, one more doctor, one more test.

At around the same time, Beth and Ben realized my mortality and became aware that the time for them to take over might be imminent. They became frustrated with me, urging me to get off Suzy's back, to stop infantilizing her. I heard their words but could not change my behavior. They had both had to give so much patience and tolerance through the years to situations where Suzy might not have used filters, and I respected the kindness and compassion they exuded but also understood the toll it had taken on their own lives. When you have a special-needs child, fair is just not equal and the impact on the siblings is significant.

After Al semiretired, both Ben and Beth urged me to pay more attention to my marriage, to spoiling my husband and giving him what he needed to have some pleasure late in his life. I tried, I really did, but I could not let go of my responsibility to Suzy to ensure that I would not let one opportunity go unexplored for finding a solution to her illnesses.

Raising Suzy was a personal battle for me, as I faced criticism from others. People intervened without being asked, which made me defensive and angry. Many failed to understand our relationship and my only response to them was, "You have not walked in my shoes or felt the pavement beneath them." I have told those who judged me that I derived self-respect and happiness by being an advocate for Suzy in all her battles. Clearly my identity was wrapped up in hers, but I have never felt any resentment towards her. My vision was clear from day one, and that was to speak out on Suzy's behalf and for her benefit, never for myself.

I always preferred to describe us as symbiotic—a mutually beneficial relationship between two people. Suzy depended on me, and I depended on her—for help, hope, purpose. I was not a martyr. I was a devoted mother.

Before Suzy's health crises, I was able to create an environment for her that fostered her independence and self-esteem. Our extended family safety net has given her the courage to survive the tremendous obstacles that she has faced throughout her life. With this constant reinforcement, she has felt like the most adored woman in the world. We gave her the security to be her best self, which is what she ultimately became, and for that I am grateful to everyone who participated in nurturing her.

As Suzy's health deteriorates and I age, I think about how it will end. I could not imagine a world without Suzy, and I would not imagine a world where Suzy would live without me. Yes, I lost my independence. I compromised my identity by being unable to separate from Suzy, needing to feel that I was doing everything I possibly could to ensure her survival. I often used to say that our hearts beat as one. I was happy with that. I would have done nothing different in the way I parented Suzy. I had to make very tough decisions, and I don't regret or apologize for any of them.

Epilogue

A mother's love knows no bounds, transcending time,
distance and circumstance; it is a boundless, relentless force
that illuminates the deepest corners of our hearts.
—SOURCE UNKNOWN

Telling Suzy's amazing story represents the fruition of a dream for me as her mother—a dream to share Suzy's story with the world. But the larger dream come true will return to Suzy herself as she comes to know that her difficult life, in all of its complex dimensions, shall be both validated and memorialized through the gifts she leaves to the world.

Yes, I hope the book has allowed you to understand what her life has been like as a neurologically impaired human being, compounded by a myriad of serious medical issues—a journey spanning forty-nine years of both struggle and triumph on all levels.

My hope, however, goes far deeper—deeper than her limitations, deeper than her initial prognoses, deeper than her adjustments, her fears, her courage, her accomplishments, her hopes, her aspirations. While those variables are all central to her story, there is a stronger, fundamental core, a fountainhead, that speaks to the very fiber of her being and above all else, defines the real reason why her story matters, why it breathes, why it had to be told and live on. It is found in the way Suzy touches and influences the lives of others, whomever she meets: leaving them better than the way they were before, leaving them to consider how they may make a difference, leaving them more hopeful, more insightful, more inclined to respond to their better angels, kinder, bolder, because one Suzy Fischer showed them the way through the gentle, pure, and loving power of her own example.

That may be the force that places her in a league of her own among those who are born into the difficult web of neurological disabilities and medical conditions. It lies not in the nature or severity of the disabilities themselves or even the way they manifest, but rather the way she works with them and within them and manages to get outside of herself and embrace others: prominent doctors, educators, members of the cloth, peers, hospital staff, whoever occupies the turf on which she lands.

It is my hope that my voice has been clear enough to help readers follow her roller-coaster ride of facing life's challenges, a ride best described by the poets: "Life is not about waiting for the storms to pass. It's about learning to dance in the rain." But my greater hope is that having read her story, you, dear reader, will have felt her presence and acknowledged its meaning—that of reaching out, extending a hand, helping others to stand tall, insisting on decency, being forever kind, and always loving hard. That is who Suzy is.

It has been said that while we inhabit this world, there is nothing more important than human beings and nothing sweeter than the human touch. If that is true, Suzy affirms it every day of her life, regardless of where God asks her to travel.

For all of us, there comes a time when God calls us home. For Suzy, my hope is that this book will enable her journey to forever remain alive for others to put up a lens to the world of the disabled and to one remarkable woman—my daughter, my master teacher—who defied all the odds and never stopped making the world a more beautiful place to know just through knowing her. My prayer is for Suzy's life to continue to unfold far into the future. But when she ultimately leaves us, I know she will do so hearing the kind of tribute that only a Shakespeare can give: "May flights of angels sing thee to thy rest."

RESOURCES FOR PARENTS AND PROFESSIONALS

Here is a list of resources in the United States for people experiencing cognitive challenges, medical issues, or rare genetic syndromes. I hope that you find them helpful. I apologize for not having a more global list, but as a US citizen, I am only recommending resources that I have interacted with or know something about.

EARLY INTERVENTION
Families with developmental concerns about children under the age of three may seek assistance from the Early Intervention System.

Early Intervention System
1-888-653-4463
www.hunterdonhealth.org/services/child

PARENTAL RIGHTS IN SPECIAL EDUCATION
Comprehensive manual for Parental Rights in Special Education from Preschool through Adults.

www2.ed.gov/parents/needs/speced/iepguide/index.html

State of New Jersey Department of Education Parental Rights in Special Education (nj.gov)

Parent Guide to HIB in NJ

www.state.nj.us/education/students/safety/behavior/hib/Parent-Guide.pdf

NJAC 6A:14

www.state.nj.us/education/code/current/title6a/chap14.pdf

ASSOCIATIONS, COUNCILS, CENTERS, AND SOCIETIES

Alliance of Special Education Schools of North Jersey

Providing information to parents, educators and other professionals about the options available for children with special needs and their rights under state laws and Department of Education guidelines. www.specialeducationalliancenj.org

AUTISM SPEAKS

email: contactus@autismspeaks.org

www.autismspeaks.org

212-252-8584 New York Office

609-228-7310 Princeton Office

NATIONAL DOWN SYNDROME SOCIETY

email: info@ndss.org

www.ndss.org

800-221-4602

NAPSEC

(National Association of Private Special Education Centers) Transition Timeline. Help for your child at different stages, from age 12 through 20½.
email: napsec@aol.com
202-408-3338

Autism Society: Since 1965, the Autism Society has been providing information for individuals on the spectrum, family members, and professionals.

Council for Exceptional Children: The Council for Exceptional Children provides information and resources about Special Education.

Easter Seals: For almost 100 years, Easter Seals has been providing services to those with special needs and disabilities.

Family Voices: Children and youth with special health care needs can benefit from Family Voices.

Federation for Children with Special Needs: The focus of the Federation for Children with Special Needs is on the parents and providing support for them, which in turn benefits the child with special needs.

BELLOWS FUND (United Cerebral Palsy)
email: info@ucpncsnj.org
908-879-2243 ext. 26

BRAIN INJURY ASSOCIATION OF NEW JERSEY
email: info@bianj.org
www.bianj.org
888-285-3036

CATASTROPHIC ILLNESS IN CHILDREN RELIEF FUND
    COMMISSION (NJ Dept. of Human Services)
1-800-335-FUND (3863), 609-292-0600
www.state.nj.us/humanservices/cicrf

DISABLED CHILDREN'S RELIEF FUND
516-377-1605
website: www.dcrf.com

HEALING THE CHILDREN—Midlantic Chapter
973-949-5034
email: info@htcnj.org
website: www.htcnj.org

HEIGHTENED INDEPENDENCE & PROGRESS (HIP)*
email: ber@hipcil.org
201-996-9100 Bergen County Office
email: hud@hipcil.org
201-533-4407 Hudson County Office
www.hipcil.org

KELLY ANNE DOLAN FUND LISTING
www.kadmf.org
215-643-0763

---

* Ask about the Sail (Special Assistance for Independent Living) Program

NEIGHBORHEART (Quality of Life Grants)
www.neighborheart.pledgepage.org
267-352-4765

NEW JERSEY DIVISION OF
  DEVELOPMENTAL DISABILITIES (DDD)
The Division of Developmental Disabilities provides public funding for services and supports that assist New Jersey adults with intellectual and developmental disabilities age twenty-one and older to live as independently as possible. Services and supports are available in the community from independent providers and in five state-run developmental centers. www.state.nj.us/human services/ddd

RAINBOW FOUNDATION
email: rainbowfoundationnj@hotmail.com
www.rainbowfoundation.org
732-671-4343

SPECIAL CHILD HEALTH SERVICES
www.state.nj.us/health/fhs/sch
609-292-7837
800-367-6543 (Toll-free in NJ)

UNITEDHEALTHCARE CHILDREN'S FOUNDATION
Call and leave a message. A foundation representative will return call within five business days.
www.uhccf.org
952-992-4459

Family Resource Center on Disabilities: Training, assistance, and information are given to parents of children with disabilities by the Family Resource Center on Disabilities.

National Association of Parents with Children in Special Education (NAPCSE): Parents of Special Education students can learn how to be their child's best advocate.

Family Hope Center: When children or adults have special needs, the Family Hope Center provides support to the entire family.

Family Resource Center on Disabilities: Training, assistance, and information are given to parents of children with disabilities by the Family Resource Center on Disabilities.

National Association of Parents with Children in Special Education (NAPCSE): Parents of Special Education students can learn how to be their child's best advocate.

National Council on Independent Living: NCIL pro

National Center for Learning Disabilities: Children and adults with learning disabilities will benefit from the information and resources available from the National Center for Learning Disabilities.

National Collaborative on Workforce and Disability: NCWD for Youth provides strategies and development systems for youth with disabilities to join the workforce.

National Down Syndrome Society: The ndss supports people with Down Syndrome by providing resources such as wellness, education, and research.

Pacer Center: The Parent Advocacy Coalition for Educational Rights utilizes the idea of parents helping parents and provides support and resources for children and youth with disabilities and their families.

Parent to Parent USA: Offers support to parents of children with special needs.

United Spinal Association: The United Spinal Association offers support, advice, and resources for those with spinal cord injuries.

Center for Parent Information and Resources
c/o Statewide Parent Advocacy Network (SPAN)
570 Broad Street, Suite 702 | Newark, NJ 07102 | 973-642-8100

For immediate or emergency mental health assistance please dial 911. If you or your child are experiencing mental health concerns you should also reach out to one of the following contacts for help and/or support.

National Suicide Prevention Helpline:
Call 1-800-273-TALK (8255) at any time to be connected to a skilled, trained counselor at a crisis center.
Perform Care Mobile Response Services: 1-877-652-7624

NATIONAL ORGANIZATION FOR RARE DISORDERS (NORD)

JOUBERT SYNDROME & RELATED DISORDERS
FOUNDATION
PO Box #84
Spokane, WA 99210 US
952-240-4853

SCHOOLS, CAMPS AND POST SECONDARY OPPORTUNITIES

ASAH

This non-profit is an umbrella organization of private schools and agencies in New Jersey.
email: info@asah.org
www.asah.org. (Información disponible en español.)
www.asah.org
609-890-1400

ECLC: "Education, Careers & Lifelong Community" for
Children and Adults with Special Needs.
Principal Jason Killian
21 Lum Avenue
Chatham, N.J. 07928
email: jkillian@eclcofnj.org
973-635-1700

Maplebrook School. Maplebrook is recognized as one of America's premier coed boarding schools focused on educating students of below average cognition with neurodiverse and complex learning profiles. It is located in Amenia, New York.

email: admissions@maplebrookschool.org

Jespy House. Based in South Orange, Jespy House is a non-profit organization that has supported adults with intellectual and Developmental Disabilities for more than forty years.

email: administration@jespy.org or call 973-762-6909

CAMPS for Youngsters with Special Needs:

Information about the Summit Camp and its expansive programming opportunities for unique campers, please contact Shep at: 570-253-4381 or 917-613-1002

email: Shep@summitcamp.com

www.summitcamp.com

FINANCIAL ASSISTANCE

Financial Assistance from ASAH to learn your rights and ensure your child receives the best possible education, including the choice for a private school placement option, if appropriate. Call ASAH's Parent Assistance Line at 1-877-287-2724, for more information.

ABLE ACCOUNTS

The ABLE Act creates tax-free savings accounts for individuals with disabilities. The bill aims to ease financial strains faced by individuals with disabilities by making tax-free savings accounts available to cover qualified expenses, such as education, housing and transportation.

www.ndss.org

RESOURCES FOR TRANPLANT

UNOS.org. The United Network For Organ Sharing is a non-profit scientific and Educational organization that administers the only organ procurement and Transplantation network in the United States. It was established by the US Congress in 1984.

LifeLink Foundation. A non-profit community service organization dedicated to the recovery of life-saving and life-enhancing organs and tissue for transplantation therapy.

National Kidney Foundation. A non-profit health organization dedicated to preventing kidney and urinary tract diseases, improving the health and well-being of individuals and families affected by kidney disease and increasing the availability of all organs for transplantation.

Putting Patients First. An initiative launched by the National Health Council to connect people living with chronic diseases and disabilities to resources and organizations focused on their particular needs.

Transplant Living Web Site. Patient-oriented website providing information on what happens before and after transplant.

United Network for Organ Sharing (UNOS). The private, non-profit organization that manages the nation's organ transplant system under contract with the federal government

Organ Procurement and Transplantation Network (OPTN). The OPTN is a public-private partnership that links all professionals involved in the US organ donation and transplantation system.

organdonor.gov. The website for the Health Resources and Services Administration (HRSA) of the US Department of Health and Human Services, information about organ donation.

ConsumerAffairs.com. This online pharmacy website provides reviews, brand comparisons, and features on various online pharmacies.

Opportunities for Organ Donor Intervention Research. Infographic that includes the steps involved in organ donation and transplantation.

UNOS Parent Guide: A comprehensive guide for parents that have children facing transplantation.

Pediatric Kidney Transplantation: A guide for patients and families that have a child facing a kidney transplant.

ACKNOWLEDGMENTS

I am certain Suzy would agree that her story would be very different without the love and support of so many wonderful, caring family members, friends, and professionals. While it is impossible to name everyone, I would like to mention a few.

To my children Ben and Beth, who have been mainstays in Suzy's development and all levels of her life. You always believed in Suzy and taught her to believe in herself—not by teaching and coaching for hours on end, but by loving her 24/7. You gave Suzy motivation to believe that excuses were unacceptable and never allowed anyone to dismiss her. You embraced her abilities as she fought her disabilities. Thank you both for being Suzy's life mentors whose love and friendship she will always cherish and hold dear.

Beth's daughters, Sydney and Alyssa Rubin and Ben's son and daughter Cole and Bailey have loved their "special Aunt Suzy" through the incredible example of their parents. Suzy, in turn adores them all and her greatest joy is spoiling them. In addition, Beth and Ben chose wonderful spouses and significant others, Britt, Bart and Lee, who have brought her continued love and support.

My eternal gratitude goes to my brothers, Marc and Neal, both doctors themselves, whose guidance, expertise, and unrelenting advice and direction in navigating Suzy's journey have been my lifeline. Their extended families, Mona, Judy, and their children have created a tribe that Suzy has always considered her own and provided structure for a sense of belonging.

Mom, you were my rock and my role model for motherhood. I miss you every day, especially your gentle soothing when I feel like life is out of control. Love doesn't describe what you mean to me.

To all the doctors, therapists, nurses, teachers, and friends who have become the fierce, determined individuals of Team Suzy, our gratitude is limitless. Although there are too many of you to mention by name, you know who you are, and there are simply no words to express our love and appreciation for all you have done. As Suzy so appropriately stated to each one of you, "Thanks you so much for putting up with my mother and all her questions. She means well, but she only bothers you so much because she loves me so much."

This book would not be possible without Carol Ann Ross who listened to my tales and so beautifully helped me put them on the pages, and Ellen Goldberg, who brought the book to Gilles Dana, publisher of G&D media, who so graciously agreed to bring it to the world with the help of his wonderful staff, including Meghan Day Healey who so patiently made all our corrections and changes and beautifully designed the interior of our book; and David Rheinhardt who designed a beautiful cover. You have all given me limitless amount of your time, and I will be forever grateful for all your guidance, keeping me on track, pushing me to be succinct, and most of all, enabling me to share the story of my most precious Suzy with the universe. Also, five other special people,

Tony and Sharon Toriello, Linda Halperin, Lynn Deutsch, and Neil Prupis, have been our champions and cheerleaders in the writing of this story.

Last, but not least, I want to acknowledge and thank my husband, Al. Al remains the Trojan horse and whatever needs go unmet for him because of my "style" of mothering, his commitment to Suzy and our entire family is unwavering. We continue to survive each crisis because of our fierce loyalty and devotion to each other and the presence of a very special child named Suzy, who shakes our world with many multifaceted complications, but at the same time, brings us light and a special breed of love.

ABOUT THE AUTHORS

JANE FISCHER, MA, LEARNING CONSULTANT

Jane Fischer became a Special Education Professional, Teacher of the Handicapped, and Learning Consultant after giving birth to a child with severe neurological deficiencies. Jane has served as an advocate for thousands of other special needs children and their families.

An active member of many local and broad-based communities, Jane serves or has served on myriad committees for special needs children. An exhaustive list includes the Board of Trustees of Early Childhood Learning Center (ECLC), a school for children with disabilities. Jane was the Founder and Inaugural President of Livingston, New Jersey's, special education PTA, Parents and Professional for Exceptional Children (PPEC).

In addition to her work as a parent and learning consultant, Jane has volunteered at the bureaucratic level for decades. With UNOS, the United Network for Organ Sharing, Jane and Suzy helped educate and guide others facing medical challenges in the unfamiliar world of organ and tissue donation. Jane and Suzy's efforts around organ donation have provided the impetus for the Essex County government to participate in a national program to honor awareness about organ and tissue donation. Also, as a leader in the Joubert Syndrome Parent Support Group, Jane and Suzy are essential resources to the researchers at the University of Washington School of Medicine in the Developmental-Behavioral Department, the Department of Pediatrics, Center for Integrative Brain Research, and the Seattle Children's Research Institute.

CAROL ANN ROSS was raised in South Africa by a literature professor who taught her to read at the age of two. After leaving South Africa due to the political unrest, Carol Ann worked as an au pair in London, a model in Paris, a GO at Club Med, studied Fashion Merchandising in Los Angeles, and ultimately became a wife, and mother to four babies. After moving to New York City, she returned to school to study Forensic Psychology, but her catering and event planning company took too much of her attention and she enjoyed a long career planning extraordinary events worldwide. During these years, she was also commissioned as a speechwriter and travel blogger.

Carol Ann served on several boards in New York, including Family Dynamics, a foundation endeavoring to keep vulnerable families together. She created her own 501c (3) called Association to Benefit Children, which provided services to children living in homeless shelters. She has been a lifetime volunteer both in the US and around the world, developing programs to lift up at risk communities.

In 2020, after moving to Miami, Carol Ann became an ordained life minister and has created unique and personal wedding ceremonies for many clients. Her wedding officiant services have taken her to many unique destinations.

If you knew Suzy is her first published work.

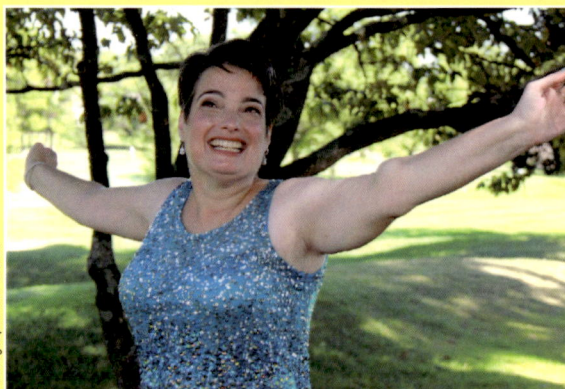

"Do not go where the path may lead, go instead where there is no path and leave a trail."

—RALPH WALDO EMERSON

Born with severe brain defects, Suzy was sentenced to a life of "nevers." With the unwavering support of her mother, Jane, and extended family, Suzy's miraculous journey has given many experts reason to question the medical textbooks that have been written. From predictions that she would never walk, talk, or function in society, Suzy overcame all these obstacles with determination and perseverance—not even allowing final-stage renal failure at the age of twenty-four to deter her. This book is not just a tribute to Suzy, but a roadmap for all parents experiencing the challenges of raising a child with disabilities and/or medical issues.

Never a victim, Suzy proceeded through infant stimulation, studies in public and specialized schools, and summer programs geared to the disabled community. Her achievements include winning medals during the Tournament of Champions, performing in a dance recital, celebrating a Bat Mitzvah, living independently, and holding a position as a classroom assistant for the past twenty-three years. Her joy of life to this day, offers us hope while showing us that giving up is not a choice.

While her IQ score identifies Suzy with severe intellectual disabilities, she never ceases to show kindness, empathy, selflessness, and compassion for others. Told with the hope that other parents will learn from her successes, and failures, this is also a story of the power of perseverance, courage, and love.

ISBN 978-1-7225-0710-7

9 781722 507107

90000

G&D MEDIA

Published by
Gildan Media LLC
aka G&D Media
www.GandDmedia.com

Endorsements for *If You Knew Suzy*

"Jane Fischer has captured the essence of meeting the challenges of parenting a child with developmental disabilities. *If You Knew Suzy* is a compassionate and instructive portrayal. It should be required reading for parents and professionals responsible for shaping such lives."

—WARREN E. HEISS, Ed.D. Professor Emeritus, Former Chair, Department of Communication Sciences and Disorders Montclair State University

"*If You Knew Suzy* is a poignant account of how a mother's love and advocacy can positively influence the life of a child with even the most dire of medical predictions. A must-read for any family starting their journey with a child with special needs."

—JENNIFER C. DEMPSEY, MPH Research Coordinator, Hindbrain Malformation Research Program at the University of Washington

"Suzy Fischer has defied all the books I have read as well as written. She is a miracle."

—ARNOLD GOLD, M.D., Former Professor of Clinical Neurology and Pediatrics, College of Physicians and Surgeons, Columbia University

"May the Suzy Effect, as described in this book, inspire every family to enjoy and love each of their children with new appreciation and joy, especially children like Suzy, whose potential is impossible to accurately forecast."

—DR. SANDRA O. GOLD MMS, EdD, Co-Founder and Trustee of the Arnold P. Gold Foundation, the leading national nonprofit championing humanism in healthcare.

"Suzy's story will encourage readers to reassess what they think of as misfortune—especially parents with any type of challenge. This story will motivate families to accept that while life hasn't gone according to plan, it has presented the unexpected blessings of new gifts, deeper experiences, and rewards."

—KATHLEEN GRISSOM, *New York Times* bestselling author of *The Kitchen House*; *Glory Over Everything* and *Crow Mary: A Novel*

"I loved this story of a determined mother, an even more determined daughter, and the family that rallied around them. Jane Fischer doesn't pull any punches describing decisions she made that she now feels

weren't the best at the time. . . . her honest account of the challenges of raising a child who has defied the medical odds is a chronicle of hope for all of us."
—MARY SIMSES, Author of The Wedding Thief

"I cannot begin to understand the journey starting the day Suzy was born. As the mother of a special needs woman, too, now age thirty-six, I have had quite a taste of it, but nothing like the years Jane has spent teaching and watching her daughter grow up as a determined and smart woman who stole the hearts of everyone she's met. I loved this book. The skilled writing gave me an exceptional understanding of not just Suzy, but of Jane and Suzy's relationship. . . . You are all heroes in my book.
—TERRY MATLEN, MSW, psychotherapist, consultant, coach, author of The Queen of Distraction and Survival Tips for Women with ADHD and founder of addconsults.com

"If you knew Suzy is a must read for anyone who has a relationship with a child with a disability. This book details the most candid, personal, and intimate experiences of a family beginning and enduring a most unexpected journey. It will serve as a roadmap to what one may expect when they are given a disability diagnosis for their child. . . . This book will help you access the courage and fortitude you will need to move forward in your journey—strengths you might not even know you possess—which will result in the best outcome possible for your child!

This book will show you some of the joys in the journey despite all the trials and tribulations—and also show you that with true grit and determination, you will survive and prevail!
—BRUCE LITINGER, Special Education Parent Advocate;
Former public school Director of Special Education;
Former Director of Approved Private Schools for Students With Disabilities

"If You Knew Suzy is an inspirational, motivational story about an incredible young lady who conquered so many challenges. As one of her many doctors, I have watched her struggle to overcome numerous medical issues, but her spirit, resolution, and beautiful smile never falter. Suzy's story reminds me of why I became a doctor."
—DR. RYAN GOLDBERG, Nephrologist,
Renal and Pancreas Transplant Division